A Beautiful Smile

A journey with my mother

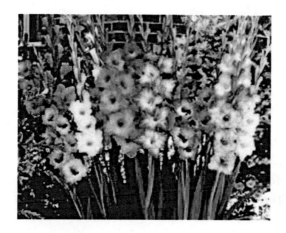

Every summer she waited patiently for our
friends Gladiolus patch to bloom with beauty,
she knew those beautiful flowers would be in a
vase on the table throughout summer

Written with love for my mother
Sandra Donalds

Chapter 1
Why I Wrote This Book?

When Mom started having unusual medical symptoms I began researching the internet and purchased a few books to learn about ALS, as well as many other neuromuscular diseases. After reviewing the books I bought, I felt like I needed more information and wanted something that would help answer all my questions, fears, and anxieties that related to these diseases, as well as caring for someone with a neuromuscular disease.

I soon discovered that what I wanted more than anything was to hear about the personal side with information on what to do when you are faced with this disease. It was then and there that I decided to document our journey. I didn't know where I would be going with it but I knew I would be able to help someone at sometime in the future.

This book is intended to help you understand the disease, what you can do to help, how to care for someone, and how to help yourself along the way. It was a complete surprise to our family when my Mom was diagnosed with ALS.

I read every piece of material I could get my hands on in order to help me understand the disease and how I could help care for her. This book will help you with everything from the beginning stages of emotional shock to preparing for the end of life.

There are so many people that I want to thank for supporting me during the time I cared for my Mom. They have been there for me every step of the way; during her illness, to the time she passed away, the months following her death and the encouragement they've given me to document my journal into a book.

My Husband Paul: I left our home for two to five days a week for eight months to help care for Mom and he never complained once. He hugged me when I needed it and supported me throughout her illness and the months after. He had cared for his Mother years before and understood the bond that Mom and I had. Thank you so much for comforting me when I needed it and encouraging me to stay strong for the family.

My Dad: Thank you for loving Mom for over 60 years and providing strength to the family in the last year of Mom's life. You cared for Mom with such love and respect that she was able to live out her life with dignity. She loved you with all her heart. I thank you from the bottom of my heart for the love and support you have given me.

My Daughter Crystal lives near me and, even though she has a husband and three children, has always been there for me to lean on. Whenever I would be looking out into space or having tears run down my face she always knew what to say or do to help me feel better.

My Daughter Jessica also has a husband and three children. She lives a few thousand miles away from me but I knew I could count on her call everyday at 11:00am. I would cry, laugh, worry about Mom, and cry more and she would listen, cry, laugh and talk to me until I felt better.

My Grandchildren: For giving me joy and laughter, you are the light of my life and I love all seven of you!

My friends Lynn, Ginger and Patty: Thank you for reading my book and providing valuable feedback. I couldn't have gotten through this without your support, hugs and kind words.

My friends Marcia and Barbara: You have helped me through this past year more than you can ever imagine. You were a phone call or email away and I could always count on you to comfort me when I needed it. You gave me guidance from your previous experiences and I appreciated every guiding step.

Book Reviews:

I couldn't put this book down. Ms. Donalds turned the journal
she kept while caring for her mother into a guide to help
others with ALS. Actually, she created a heartbreaking,
gripping novel that is easy to read. A journey that is sad and
funny but always informative. I recommend it to everyone,
especially those families who've received this diagnosis of a
loved one. It is an unsparingly honest, thoughtful, moving,
and informative story.
Lynn Ellen Metker
Writer, Reader
South Carolina

Sandy's book is a very personal journey in dealing in a
positive, loving and helpful way through a very difficult time.
All of the emotions, experiences and helpful information that
she expresses in this wonderfully touching story will be of
great help to others that face dealing with the awful disease
of ALS.
She does an excellent job of helping one to understand this
disease with invaluable information and helpful insights and
shines a light on what it takes to successfully walk this
difficult path in caring for a loved one who has been afflicted
with this disease.
I was captivated from the very beginning with her very
personal story and couldn't put it down and recommend it to
everyone. Not only to those dealing with ALS, but as a
source of encouragement to anyone going through a difficult
life challenge
Ginger Rea
Colleague

A life well lived...that is the impression you will have when you finish this book. Shirley Gearhart lived her life for others, and took great joy in each moment. Her daughter, Sandy, has written a journal to honor her mother; it's a good book for this reason alone. But the valuable information on dealing with a terminal illness in a loved one will help countless individuals who are in the same position. Read this book for a picture of family love. And read it for its practical information, as well. You will learn how to help your loved one in so many ways – making them physically comfortable, maintaining their dignity, ensuring that they feel loved and safe at all times. And you'll learn about the help that is available from agencies like Medicare and Hospice. And finally, you will get to know Sandy – a very special lady who learned to love from her mother. One that I can love as well!

Patty Fultz
Avid Reader, Missionary
Brazil

Every year an estimated 5,600 Americans are diagnosed with ALS.

It is one of the most common neuromuscular diseases worldwide, and as many as 30,000 Americans have ALS.

www.alsa.org
The ALS Association website

Definition: Amyotrophic Lateral Sclerosis (ALS) is a neurological disease of the motor neurons; muscle-controlling nerve cells in the brain and spinal cord that control voluntary muscle movement. The neurons are an important communication link between the nervous system and the voluntary muscles. As the motor neurons break down and die they stop transmitting messages to the muscles and the patient eventually loses all control of their muscles.

ALS does not affect the ability to smell, taste, hear, or see, and patients normally maintain control of eye muscles and bladder/ bowel functions.

Cause: Generally unknown, motor neurons prematurely degenerate and die. Genetic factors are thought to play a 10% role with a family history.

Onset: Usually adulthood, the normal age is 40-50 but my Mom was diagnosed at the age of 75.

Symptoms: Generalized weakness and decrease use of muscles as well as some muscle cramping and muscle twitching.

Progression: ALS affects the voluntary muscles of the upper and lower body including the legs, arms, throat, and mouth muscles. This disease will ultimately affect all voluntary muscles resulting in paralysis. Usual survival rate averages three to five years although it will be different in every situation, as some people have been known to only live one year or less.

There isn't any way of knowing exactly how long the patient will live and I recommend you begin preparing your family for the end of life within the first few months of learning of the disease, especially if the patient is older than 65. Mom was 75 and died within nine months of the diagnosis.

Insurance:

www.medicare.gov

Medicare covers ALS, regardless of age

If you have ALS (Amyotrophic Lateral Sclerosis, also called Lou Gehrig's disease), you automatically are approved for Part A and Part B the month your disability benefits begin.

You must have a series of medical tests completed including the nerve conduction studies that your neurologist will order. This is the only disease that Medicare approves coverage immediately. If you have insurance through your employer, keep it active so that it can pick up the balance that Medicare doesn't pay.

Once Hospice becomes involved, they will bill Medicare and your portion of the balance should be minimal if any at all.

Social Security Benefits:

www.socialsecurity-disability.org

This particular disease is contained in the listing of disabling medical conditions covered under the SSA's Compassionate Allowances program. Because of this, individuals who apply for disability benefits due to a case of Amyotrophic Lateral Sclerosis are often able to be approved for benefits in less than a month.

A definite diagnosis of ALS (amyotrophic lateral sclerosis) disease is needed to secure SSA disability benefits. Other factors such as age, education, past relevant work and/or residual functional capacity are not considered.

Hospice:

www.hospicenet.org

Hospice is there to help you and your family with the medical and emotional needs that arise during the course of this disease. With the help of Hospice we were able to keep Mom at home for the duration of her disease and she died peacefully with her family by her side.

Make a contact with the local Hospice association to inform them of the disease and ask them if and when they would become involved. Once they became involved they took care of all equipment, supplies and medicine needs. Your Hospice team may work differently in your area so check with them as early as possible to determine how they will assist you.

Chapter 2
The Signs and Symptoms

Summer 2009:

Mom tells me she doesn't understand why she is so tired and weak, and that she is having trouble doing anything for more than a few minutes without having to rest. She can't describe it and says it's nothing like she's ever experienced and it's a different kind of weakness. I say, "Mom, you work too hard and worry too much about keeping the house spotless so just rest when you get tired and don't worry so much."

I didn't think much about it at the time. She is seventy-five and it's normal to start tiring a little easier as you age. As the summer goes on she is so tired all the time and it begins to concern me. My Mom and Dad do not live near any of their children and I've always wondered what would happen if my parent's got sick.

Now I think it's time to really start considering what we would do. I have one brother that lives with my parent's, a sister lives three hours away in Pittsburgh, my oldest brother lives in California, my youngest brother lives in Las Vegas and I live in Ohio where my parents live, but about an hour away. I see my parents more than any of the other siblings and she's very comfortable around my husband and me.

My parents live near a beautiful lake and we would normally visit their house quite often during the summer, as did many relatives and friends. My sister and I talk on the phone often and discuss our concern with Mom being so tired all the time. We know that she cleans the house for days when someone is planning to visit and it's sad to think how tired she gets cleaning the house. We think about not visiting as much but that wouldn't help any of us since we love seeing our parents. There's no need for Mom to worry so much about the house when we visit so we think about just not telling her when we plan to visit. That she wouldn't use all her energy to clean the house before we got there. Her house is always so clean that you could probably eat off her floors but she still worries when someone is visiting and puts extra effort into cleaning, even when it's us! It wears her out when she knows someone is coming for a visit.

If Mom has one thing that bothers us it's how she worries about keeping the house clean but that's what makes her happy, a clean, clean house! Funny though, my daughters said the same thing about me when they were younger! Now I'm thinking *"If I'm like my Mom then I am honored."*

I should have started concerning myself with Mom when my husband and I visited in our motor home. We had just purchased a motor home and took it over to their house for the weekend. Mom stepped up about two steps into the motor home and thought it would be perfect for the extra space needed when we had several people staying at their house for the weekends.

When she started walking out of the motor home onto the first step she lost her balance because she couldn't grip the handle tight enough to hold herself. She fell off the steps and landed on her side and I heard my sister scream and I ran over to her to see what happened. Thank goodness it was only a couple steps.

I sat down beside Mom on the ground and asked her if she was hurt and started to help her get up. She said in a worried voice, "I'm not hurt but I need to sit here for a few minutes before I get up." She's never fallen like this before and I didn't realize that she fell because she couldn't grip the handle. Luckily she only fell a few steps down and didn't hurt herself.

We sat on the ground for a few minutes before Mom said that she felt good enough to get up. I helped her up and we walked in the house arm in arm to make sure she was stable.

So, when we think back to that time we realize it could have been the beginning of the disease, which was a year prior to her diagnosis.

My Mom is such a nice and caring person. She has so much class and I've never heard her say negative remarks about anyone. She was the one in the family that kept the peace. Sure she had her disagreements with family members but she would always look for the good side in everyone.

I admired her when I was a young adult stressed about work and raising children and she always remained calm. I would think, "How does she do that. Nothing bothers her." What a great person my Mom is! She is such a terrific wife, mother, grandmother, sister, aunt, and friend.

Mom never complains about anything but throughout the summer and autumn she would tell me she was so tired and couldn't understand why. She wasn't doing anything different but she just didn't have any energy and her body felt different. I kept telling her that she works too hard and to take it easy.

Again, I didn't think much about it other than she's starting to get older. I have learned so much from my Mom during my lifetime, and the one thing that continues to stick out is to take it one day at a time and to not worry about the things you can't change. One of her famous quotes that I live by today is: "It is what it is." Anytime something would happen she would say that we can't change it and will do what we can to move forward. Wow, was that a statement that would come so true during the next year!

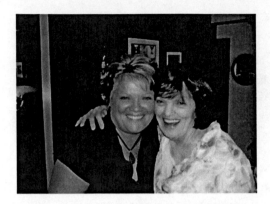

Mom and I at my daughter's baby shower in
August, 2009.
She has such a beautiful smile.

November and December 2009:

Mom and Dad always come to our house for the holidays, as does my sister, her family, my daughters, their families, my husband's children, and their families. The holidays are such a wonderful time for us. There is so much love and laughter in our home during the holidays. Cooking together, laughing and cleaning up. Once everything is put away all of us girls take a trip to the local discount stores. We never need anything but always have a good time shopping around together and laughing.

Mom is healthy and looking good. She's so beautiful. I am always taking pictures and this year is no different. I post a few on Face Book and so many of our old friends and neighbors comment about how great Mom looks and how beautiful her smile is. I agree and say, "I know I hope I look as good as she does at 75."

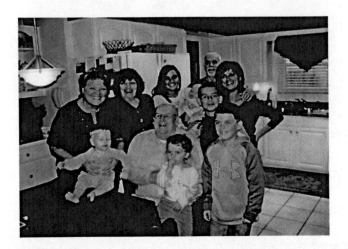

December 2009, all smiles, the holidays were wonderful this year with Mom (second from left in back) and Dad (second from left in front). If I only knew then that it would be the last holiday with Mom as a healthy, strong woman.

February and March 2010:

Mom starts to tell me that something is wrong with her left arm because it's losing strength and she can't use it very well. It doesn't hurt but she doesn't understand what is wrong. I ask her if she has any other symptoms; thinking she may have had a small stroke.

I haven't seen her since Christmas so I'm not able to see if she has any visible signs of a stroke. But nothing else seems to be wrong other than being tired and her left arm getting weak. I call more often to see how she is and ask her to see her doctor. She said she has a routine appointment coming up and will ask the doctor about it then. It concerns me that she is so tired all the time and weaker than she should be.

Dad likes to take Mom to the casino to play the slot machines every other week or so. They aren't using any money that they don't have and I think it's great that they have so much fun together. Mom begins to tell me that she gets so tired when they go and they don't stay as long anymore. When Mom is going home early from their fun times I know something is wrong. I keep asking her if she has seen her doctor but she says she is just going to wait until her routine appointment. I talk to my Dad about wanting Mom to see her doctor and he does say that he can see she's tired more than normal and is beginning to worry about her also. I ask him to try to get her to the doctor soon.

April 2010:

My daughter moves into her new house and decides that she will take over the holiday dinners. Her house can hold a large group of people and she's about the age I was when I took over the dinners, so I guess it is time!

She holds the Easter dinner with our family and her husband's family. Mom looks good but I can see that she isn't able to use her left arm. It really hit my daughter when her grandma couldn't hold her baby. When my daughter offered the baby to Mom she said, "I don't think I can hold him because my arm doesn't have any strength in it and I don't want to drop him."

My daughter's heart broke because she had no idea Mom was that bad. Mom told me later that she felt terrible for my daughter and I told her she shouldn't worry about it. We have a really good time but I can see that Mom is getting tired so we don't stay very late. We come to my house and she rests for awhile.

- **Mom shows me her arm, it's swollen from not being used and she can't touch her fingers to her thumb. Her fingers are starting to curl and she keeps pressing them flat on the table, hoping that it will straighten out on its own.**

It's hard to believe that Mom was healthy a few months ago.

I keep asking her if anything else is wrong and she says that it's only her arm and that her body feels tired all the time. She doesn't understand why she's so tired. I ask her to not wait any longer to see the doctor and she says she will call as soon as they get home. I'm feeling it may be serious and it breaks my heart to see this happening to her.

Dad isn't in great health. He has a bad back and knee and he's not as secure on his feet as he used to be. I worry about Mom's health getting worse while Dad already has these few health issues. At 75 and 78, they have been enjoying their retirement and family to the fullest and it breaks my heart that things are beginning to change.

Mom and Dad finally go to the doctor between Easter and Mother's Day.   Mom has blood work done twice and X-rays of her arm, wrist and hand. All blood work comes back normal and the doctor says she probably has a rotator cuff tear and arthritis of her wrist.

What I don't understand is why her doctor says that he 'thinks' she has these problems. Shouldn't he know? I'm thinking he has a feeling it's something else and doesn't want to tell her until he knows for sure. When I talk to Mom on the phone I'm frustrated because I don't think her doctor is doing everything he can be doing to figure this out for her.

I'm concerned that it's something more serious. She had a blood clot in her leg a few years ago and they told her at that time that her heart wasn't 100%, so I'm concerned it may have something to do with her heart. My grandma had a weak heart also and that is what eventually led to her death.

- **What I eventually realized is that the Doctors were trying to rule out ALS, they just didn't want to tell us until they were sure. If you have any indication that it may be ALS go ahead and ask those questions. It's better to be prepared.**

I call Mom a few times a week to see how she's feeling. The week before Mother's Day I called and she sounded so weak that she could hardly talk. I could hardly stand listening to her talking so weak and it broke my heart to think it could be something serious. I was so sad that she was feeling so weak and was having difficulty carrying on the conversation.

I begin researching her symptoms on the internet. I had heard of ALS and watched the Lou Gehrig movie many years ago, but never in a million years would I think that Mom would be given that diagnosis. I was still thinking she probably had a small stroke and was still recovering.

She could hear my concern in my voice each time we talked on the phone and told me not to worry, that she probably just has arthritis or something like that. I told her to not worry about the house and to rest as much as she could. I told her I would clean the house when I came to visit that weekend for Mother's Day.

Mother's Day 2010:

I decide to visit Mom and Dad by myself this weekend. I wasn't sure what I would be seeing and not sure how long I would stay. My husband knew how concerned I was about Mom and I told him I may want to stay a few days longer than normal. He told me to go ahead and stay as long as I needed and he would stay home with the dogs this time.

Oh my Gosh, it took everything I had to not cry the entire time I was there! Mom is so weak and not walking very steady. This is something completely new to us. How can this happen in a matter of a few weeks? I just saw her at Easter and she was fine with the exception of being tired and not having the use of her left arm or hand.

This can't be my Mom, who just 5 months ago was walking around normal, cleaning, cooking, ironing, sweeping, washing dishes, shopping, and everything a normal healthy woman does. What is happening to my wonderful Mom? This isn't fair and I'm so sad.

I always help with the cooking and cleaning when I'm there but this time I do everything since she really isn't able to do much anymore. I also want to help Dad as much as I can. I ask Dad if he knew what was wrong and he said she just seems to be getting weaker and that he has taken over most of the housework and cooking. He isn't in great health and I'm concerned he may also become ill.

- Mom has absolutely no strength in her left arm and there are so many things she can't do anymore. Her hand is curled into a fist and she can't keep it straightened out. The initial signs of ALS are shown in weakness in certain areas of the body, normally the arms or legs. There may be muscle pain or cramps in the arms and legs. Muscle twitches may also occur but don't jump to the conclusion of ALS until you receive a diagnosis. There are several neurological diseases and all others should be ruled out before confirming ALS.

What is wrong with Mom and why can't they figure this out?

Mom and I are talking and I tell her that I would iron her clothes and she was so thrilled! You would have thought I gave her a million dollars. Anyone who knows my Mom would giggle at that! Mom was known for having a spotless house and still ironing all their clothes. *I don't even iron my own unless they absolutely need it, but I enjoy ironing hers, if nothing but helping her feel good!*

Mom and I talk about what has been happening to her and how she's so tired and can't use her arm or hand. We talk about what would happen if she her other arm went weak and how difficult it would be for Dad. I mention moving in with us down the road and she says she doesn't want to even think about that yet but will if things get any worse. We don't even know what it is yet and I'm asking her if they want to move in with us.

Mom said that moving in with us would be the last resort, but does agree that she would think about it and that she would move in with us if she had to go anywhere. I promise her that I will take care of her and never allow her to go into a nursing home if something serious happens. She knew that but I wanted to make sure.

I saw how wonderful she was with grandma when she took care of her and I want to do the same for her. Mom cared for grandma until the end and never regretted one day that was spent with her Mom.

When I get ready to leave to go home Mom says she's so much happier when I'm around. I realize that I need to visit more often. It's so difficult for me to talk about caring for her and deciding what to do if something serious is wrong. It just doesn't seem right because she's always been so healthy. I can't imagine what is going to happen if she's diagnosed with something serious. But somehow I feel that terrible news is not far off.

I'm not even a mile away when I start crying non-stop for the hour drive home. I call my daughter on the way home even though I knew I shouldn't have. I was crying but I had to talk to someone. I calmed down enough to tell her what was happening with Mom and that I didn't know what I was going to do if something serious was wrong. She's crying with me and felt so bad about her grams.

When I pull in the driveway I'm still on the phone with her and still crying. My husband came out to greet me and can't figure out why I'm crying so much. When I get myself straightened out I told him about Mom and just sobbed. I just can't get over it and I called my other daughter and cried with her too. She lives so far away and feels terrible that she can't be here to console me and to see her grams.

Both of my daughters are so sad. They can't stand to see me sad because I'm normally so happy and strong and handle most things with ease. Well, it's definitely different when it's your Mom that you love with all your heart. What I will do if it's something serious? At this point it must be very serious. Mom's health problems seem to be getting worse, much quicker than I would have ever imagined.

I told a good childhood friend of mine about what was happening with Mom and, since she knew Mom well, she asked if she could visit. Certainly! Mom loved visiting with her, talking about younger days when our Mom's would sit on the porch and watch us all play. After an hour or so I could see that Mom was getting tired so we decided to leave. When we leave my friend said she was so sorry about my Mom and told me to be strong. She had helped take care of her Mom the past few years and her Mother had passed away recently. She knew what I was about to go through. Her compassion was amazing and she's helped comfort me so much along this journey. My friend took some valuable pictures of my parents before she left.

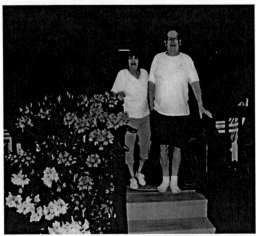

Mom and Dad in May, 2010.
She loves her flowers and is still smiling!

My Aunt, Uncle, Mom and Dad get together every week or so to play cards and UNO. After one of their recent visit my aunt calls to ask me about Mom. She sees the same things as I do and wonders what could be wrong. I don't have any answers and told her that Mom will be going back to the Doctor for more testing while they try to diagnose the problems. My aunt is so worried about Mom and tells her daughter what has been happening.

THEN all of a sudden my cousin comes across a lawsuit that seems similar to Mom's issues. She works for an attorney and she comes across a lawsuit about denture cream causing neurological problems.

MAYBE this could be it!

I search the internet and see pages of lawsuits against the company that makes denture cream. People are having neurological problems and some are even in wheelchairs because they have lost the use of their arms and legs. Oh My Gosh, could this be it? I was so excited because maybe, just maybe, we could find out what was wrong and correct it before it got too far along. It seems this problem stems from zinc and copper.

Luckily Mom had another doctor's appointment and she tells him about the information we have found. He checks the internet and found all the information he needed. He takes blood work for zinc and copper and will know something in a few days.

Mom's doctor also orders an MRI on her legs and feet to make sure her veins and muscles are healthy. She's more and more unstable when she walks and the doctor is trying to find out why. If the zinc and copper levels come back irregular that could be the problem with her back and being so unstable. We wait and hope!

- **Have Zinc and Copper levels checked, even if you don't wear dentures. Low levels could cause neurological problems.**

Well just when you think you know what could be causing the problems the results come back and slap you in the face. All of Moms blood work is normal, including the zinc and copper levels.

My poor Mom, what could she be thinking and how horrified is she? I am crying more and more these days as I think about the things that could be causing these problems. I love her so much and it pains me to think of what she is going through and I can't stand the thought of a serious health problem..

June 2010:

I'm visiting Mom and Dad and she actually seems a little better than a few weeks ago. She still has no use of her left arm and is very unstable but I think she has probably just accepted that something is wrong and is dealing with it a little better. It's not easy for any of us and I can't even imagine what Mom is feeling inside. She walks very slowly and holds onto the wall or chairs to help keep her balance.

She sitting and resting more these days and isn't able to do much because of her arm. Dad has taken over everything, including helping Mom get dressed. He always thought he would be the one that got sick and I know he never imagined this could happen to them, but he is so good with her and keeps a pretty good attitude.

I work on the ironing, cut Dad's hair and trim Mom's hair. I also got all their summer clothes out and put the winter clothes away. As I'm doing this I'm wondering if this will be the last time I help them exchange their seasonal clothes. Mom feels so much better when her clothes are all organized! I just wish I could do more. I'm beginning to realize that as time goes on I will be doing more and more for them and my heart breaks a little more as I hug them.

They are both feeling and looking a little more fragile these days.

My older brother that lives with my parents has been a blessing. He is taking care of the lawn and doing everything that needs done on the outside of the house. It's so good to know he's at the house when I'm not there, especially if something serious happened and he needed to call for help.

We have one of our grandson's graduation parties the following weekend and my sister and her family come to stay with us from Pittsburgh. Mom and Dad decided to not come to the party since Mom wasn't feeling very well, so my sister and her family stopped to visit them before coming to our house. My sister has not seen Mom since Easter and I knew she would be devastated when she saw her.

During the party my sister slides in the house and I notice that she is gone for awhile. I walk into the dining room and see her talking on the phone and I knew she was talking to Mom because she looked so sad. She is upset and gives me the phone so that I can talk to Mom.

Mom tells me that my sister can't imagine what could be wrong with her. I tell Mom that I will talk to my sister and let her know everything that has happened so far with the doctors and her health. When my sister calms down I hand the phone back to her so she could tell Mom goodbye. I knew how she felt and it broke my heart. She was devastated and I hugged her tight when she hung up. We just stood there and cried and hugged.

People walked in and around us and we really didn't notice because we were so wrapped up in our sadness and I wanted to help my sister feel safe. We each felt good getting comfort from one another. My sister was feeling the same as I did when I saw Mom on Mother's Day and her heart was broken.

It hits you like a brick and you just can't believe how someone's health can go downhill so fast. My sister had not seen Mom since Easter and this was heart wrenching for her.

She tells me that Mom is speaking a little slower, not walking stable, and not able to do much of anything. She tires easily and has to rest often. How can this be happening and how can we NOT know what is wrong yet?

I'm so glad I was here for my sister. She needed to breakdown and I held her while we both cried. As we cried we told each other that we would do anything we could to help Mom and Dad get through this. We knew the road ahead was going to be long and difficult.

Chapter 3

The Medical Testing

During the next few weeks Mom goes back to the doctor and has some nerve testing done on her legs and arms. Her Doctor refers her to a neurologist to analyze his findings and determine what is actually wrong. I secretly think he has a good idea but needs the neurologist's opinion.

Mom can't figure out why her normal doctor can't do everything and asks him why. She wants to have him figure it out. Her doctor explains that as much as he wants to, he just can't do everything and the neurologist will be able to figure it out. So she reluctantly went to the neurologist.

He ordered an MRI of her neck and spine to rule out a pinched nerve. He said there may be something in her neck that is causing the arm to lose its muscle. Mom is so frightened to get an MRI. She gets claustrophobic and is afraid that she won't make it through the test. They explain that it will be an open MRI and she shouldn't feel closed in. They even allow Dad to take her to the outpatient center to see how it's done before she schedules her own.

She reluctantly went to get the MRI and tells me about it later. She said the noise was worse than the test. It made a loud banging noise like she was in a chamber and it was so loud that it kept her mind off the MRI and she got through it just fine.

We are hoping the MRI shows that Mom has a pinched nerve and it can be fixed! Pray, pray, pray that this is it. Wouldn't that be great? Could it actually be possible that all these problems are caused by a pinched nerve?

A week later, we feel like we've been slapped again.

Everything is fine with her neck and spine and no pinched nerve. Once again we are sad and need to figure out what is wrong with Mom. It really could be something serious. The neurologist schedules nerve and muscle testing at the hospital near our home and I offered to take Mom for the tests.

I'm thinking more and more about them moving in with us.   There is no way Dad can continue to take care of Mom and everything else that needs done around the home.

Mom and Dad come over around noon on the day of her test so that I can take Mom for the testing at the hospital. Normally they would come over the day before and stay all night but Mom really doesn't want to. Since it takes her so long to get ready to go anywhere she didn't want to get ready one day to come to my house and then have to get ready the next day to go to the hospital.

I understood exactly what she meant. Mom always looks 100% when she goes out. She wants her make-up done, hair looking nice, and clothes ironed! I agree and tell her to just come early on the day of the test and we'll go from there.

We get to the hospital and Mom holds on to me very tightly while walking close to my side so that I can guide her. We are walking very slowly and she says it reminds her of the times she did the same thing with her Mom. She said she would just hold on to Grandma and pull her along. She always giggles when she thinks about her Mom. She loved her dearly, as I love her.

Mom is much slower these days and I think to myself that this can't be happening. I am so heartbroken.

We walk very slowly into the hospital and luckily the outpatient testing center isn't too far. She should be using a cane by now but doesn't want to.

- **Start using a cane or walker as soon as walking is unstable, even if you don't have a diagnosis yet.**

Having nerve and muscle testing ended up being one of the worst days of my life, not to mention my Mother's. The nerve and muscle testing took over two hours and I stayed in the room with Mom the whole time. The doctor's hooked her up to a machine so that they could watch how her nerves and muscles moved.

It was horrible watching her get small shocks to her arms and legs to see how her nerves worked, in addition to the hundreds of small needles in her muscles. My Mom is one of the strongest women I know and she rarely lets anyone see her cry.

The doctors are testing her nerves with little electric shocks all over her arms, legs, and back while watching the read-out on a machine similar to an EKG. There are two of them and they talk very quietly between themselves so that we can't hear what they are saying. I'm sitting behind them and try to figure out what the machine is saying.

I have no medical background other than working for medical insurance for thirty years, so I have just enough knowledge to be dangerous!

Then they begin the muscle testing. Same machine just louder noises. As the muscles contract the lines on the machine go crazy, up, down, up, down, up, down. It looks like a lie detector test but louder. Mom is getting frustrated and I can't blame her; lie on your back, relax, turn to your stomach, relax, relax, relax, needles poking into her EVERYWHERE, relax, move your chin down to your chest, relax, lift your arm, relax, relax, relax, curl up like a cat, relax, make your legs go up to your stomach, relax, relax, turn to your side, relax, lay your legs straight, relax, relax, relax!

Oh my Gosh, Mom starts crying!

She NEVER cries. She's my Mom. What should I do? My heart breaks. I want to scream at them for hurting her. The doctors apologize to her and tell her she's doing fine. They try to be sympathetic but they *are* doctors and they just need their information.

I wipe my tears so Mom doesn't see me crying then take some tissue over to her. She says she is so sorry for crying and the doctors tell her she's doing terrific and they really didn't mean to upset her. I tell them her left shoulder is very painful when she moves around and to please be careful. She's crying softly and it's just killing me. I'm so sad for her and want to help her.

One of the doctors tries to get her to relax by asking her about her husband and children. *WELL, that didn't go over very well.* It just made her sadder and she cried more. I was heartbroken and wondering how I was going to be strong for her.

At my age of 55, I'm a little emotional these days also! I ask Mom if she wants me to stand by her and she said that she would be ok. I reluctantly go back to my chair and sit and watch. The doctors are patient with her and very slowly get her to relax and begin the needle testing again.

My GOSH, this has been going on for 2 hours. How much do they need and how many times are they going to whisper while we are right there with them?

It's almost too much for me but I stay strong because I know it's what they need to help them make a diagnosis. I'm really beginning to worry about what they are going to tell us.

FINALLY, after another half hour, they say that she's done and start talking about their findings. The doctors ask her if she knows why she is there and she said that her doctor wanted to rule out everything. She really didn't have very much information. They start talking about ALS and ask **her if she knows what ALS is. She says "yyyyeeeeesssss, I know what it is."** If you know my Mom, you can actually hear her say this!

They say she may want to come in again to visit the hospital neurologist to get further testing and I ask, "Why?" I feel that they have done enough and should have the information they need and there isn't any reason she should have to go through this again.

Anyway, they continue talking about ALS but can't give us a definite diagnosis. They say they will send their findings to her neurologist and tell me "If it was one of my relatives, I would be extremely worried." *REALLY, I'm pretty sure you just told me the diagnosis. She has ALS.*

We thanked them and they told Mom she could get dressed and they wished us luck. OK what do we do now? I go over to Mom and hug her. She starts crying again and can't quit sobbing.

I hold her, rub her back, and keep telling her that she did great and it's all over. Holding her feels like talking to my child and it's breaking my heart while I'm trying to comfort her. She says she was sorry she just couldn't relax like they wanted her to. I tell her she shouldn't worry about being upset. The doctors got what they needed. I tell her that I doubt anyone could relax when they are being poked with hundreds of needles. She smiles a little and we go on.

I'm feeling more and more like *her Mom* these days. She was completely exhausted. I just kept hugging her and rubbing her back.

Another moment, she was beginning to feel like my child while I comforted her. I'm so sad and kept thinking to myself that I have to stay strong. I HAVE to be the strong one for this family.

We get her dressed and ready to leave. We found our way out and we were on our own, so sad and so lonely. I have never felt so alone in my life with my Mom on my arm walking slowly through the hospital. I have this sad feeling that she is very, very ill. I'm wondering how much time we will have with our Mom. I finally get her to the car and she is physically and emotionally exhausted.

We secretly know she has ALS and she says, "Please don't ever make me take a test like that again. I will never go. It doesn't matter what the doctors need." She doesn't care if there are five different doctors asking for the test. "I promise and I don't blame you. They should have everything they need anyway," I say sadly.

We talk a little about the testing but she's so tired I just quit talking and let her fall asleep on the drive home. When we get home we told my husband and Dad about the experience and again Mom asked us to never make her take any more testing of that nature. I look into Dad's eyes and they are so sad.

Chapter 4

The Diagnosis

July 2010:

It's been over a week since Mom had the nerve testing done at the hospital and she asks me to take her to the neurologist to get her diagnosis. Dad said that he would take Mom but we told him he could stay home and relax for awhile.

Mom is comfortable around me and I do all I can to comfort her. I know she keeps thinking back to the time she took care of her Mom and is comforted knowing that I will always take care of her in the same way. We drive quietly for a half hour to the neurologist's office. We secretly know this could be the last hour before the end of her healthy, safe life.

She wants to walk into the doctor's office so I have her hold on to my arm and we walk in very slowly. It takes quite awhile since she's very unstable these days. When we get into the lobby the receptionist asks if we want a wheelchair and I look at Mom knowing she really doesn't want to. She needs one and I say, "Mom, It won't be bad and you really should try," and she finally says, "OK I will try it."

This was the first time I walked anyone in a wheelchair. I thought I would have a little fun with her and bumped into a few walls going down the hall. I would say to people "I'm new at this!" and they would chuckle. We had help everywhere we went. People opened doors for us and would tell me the best way to navigate. The doctor's office was on the 2nd floor. I'm really glad she used a wheelchair. I said, "See how much better you feel." She was smiling and definitely agreed, because she didn't have to use all her energy to walk the halls.

- **Get a cane or walker as soon as possible, even if you don't have a diagnosis. If they are unstable while walking they need to feel more secure with a cane, walker, or even a wheelchair.**

We met with the neurologist. He asked us if the hospital told us anything and we said, "Not really, they said they would send the results to you." He said, "ALS is very difficult to diagnose and I sent you to have the muscle and nerve testing done to confirm my initial opinion." This was his second opinion. I told him I was glad he told us that because everything I read says to get a second opinion.

"I'm sorry but you do have ALS."

As much as we secretly knew, it still hurt and felt like a knife going through my chest.

I can't even imagine what Mom was thinking.

I think we handled it very well and asked a lot of questions. I asked about the Riluzole drug and he made a face which I felt wasn't a very good sign. He said, "You can take it but it normally gives you severe headaches and most people may only live for a few extra months." Well, having headaches wouldn't be worth it so Mom said, "no thanks." He told us that he can't tell how fast it will progress because everyone is different. It could be two months or ten years. We just need to work with it and prepare for the next phase.

I was nodding my head with every explanation the Doctor gave and asked several follow-up questions. He said that as her muscles deteriorate she will probably feel some cramping or twitching which is a sign that the part of the body cramping will most likely be the next to lose all muscle.

Mom then said, "She already knows just about everything there is to know. She's been reading anything she can get her hands on." Mom thinks I'm so smart!

The neurologist was very compassionate and I could see that he felt sad for Mom. He told mom to come back in six months to review her health.

When we left, I took the wheelchair out to the car so Mom wouldn't have to walk at all. I also knew that Mom would not be back for another doctor's visit, EVER! This was her death sentence and there isn't any reason to see a doctor. She confirmed my thoughts by saying, "there isn't any reason to go back to the doctor since there's nothing they can do."

On the way home we talk quietly about her health and what has happened to her up until this point. I told her I would gather some reading material to help her understand what will happen. We remembered the Lou Gehrig movie but have not heard much about the disease since then, which has been years.

It broke my heart as I explain what I knew about the disease, "It affects all the voluntary muscles of your body and each muscle will deteriorate. You will not be able to use them, similar to what is happening to your left arm." At this point I didn't feel like we needed to go into much detail. She knew there was no cure. If I talked too much more about it I knew that we would both break down and I didn't want that to happen while I was driving.

I told her she would continue to be tired and weak and should rest as much as possible.

Today was our day for answers after so many months of Doctor's visits and testing. The outcome was horrible but at least we could move forward with the care needed to help Mom through this terrible disease.

Mom loves McDonald's cheeseburgers so I told her we should stop and get one. She just smiled even though we knew Dad would be cooking dinner! We got our cheeseburgers and fries and she enjoyed them so much. She was just handed a death sentence but was still able to smile.

How does she do that?

It was so good to see her smile. I was silently praying for God to give me the strength to get through this. We talked about the cheeseburgers and the way we always got one when we went shopping the day after Thanksgiving with my daughters. My daughters always talk about grams loving her cheeseburgers from McDonalds!

We get home and I let Mom walk slowly into the house. She can still walk by herself as long as she has something to hold on to. I go into the kitchen with Dad and (another moment) said, *"She has ALS."*

I'm crying like a baby and he wraps his arms around me. I have never cried like this in front of my Dad. I may have had a few tears now and then but he has never seen me bawl like a baby. I was so sad I didn't know how I would get through this.

He's in his own pain but just keeps hugging me and saying, "Oh no, Oh no, Oh no," while trying to comfort me.

This seemed to go on forever but it was really only about three minutes. Mom comes into the house slowly and I stop crying and wipe my tears so that she doesn't see me. Dad walks over to Mom and hugs her tightly. I know he never wants to let her go. He asks, "What did the doctor say? What do we do now? What is going to happen?"

I explain as much as I knew at this point. I didn't know everything about the disease yet but had been reading any information I could find. I knew enough to help them understand what would happen. We haven't talked about this disease yet because we kept hoping we wouldn't have to.

I tell him that they may want to move in with us because he won't be able to take care of Mom full time. He's been doing it for a month or so now and it's already taking a toll on him. He doesn't really want to hear it but knows I'm right. *Mom even said, "She's right, you won't be able to do it all. It's too hard to take care of me."*

We talk quietly while I explain to Dad what the disease will do. I tell him that her muscles will eventually deteriorate and she won't have any use of her arms and legs. It will affect her swallowing, talking, and eventually her breathing.

I don't have it in me to say that she will die because her breathing muscles will stop. They know it and I'm thinking it. I'm not sure I will ever be able to actually say it. I can't believe I have to be talking about something this horrible.

This is the saddest day of our lives. I told them that everything I've read says to try and stay ahead of the disease by having equipment ready: wheelchair, handicapped bathroom, eating utensils, and so on. Our minds are spinning and we have a difficult time discussing things any further.

Dad has dinner ready but who can eat. We just ate McDonalds and our stomachs are already turning.
Mom is sitting in a chair and I hug her like a child and rub her back and then I start crying. She says, *"Don't cry, you'll make me cry."* Dad says *"I didn't think we be around for as long as we have, we really are lucky we've lived this long."* I try to laugh and say, *"But I want you to live forever!"* It was a little chuckle that got us through even though our hearts were broken.

We all calm down and I hug Dad again. I told them that I would call my brothers, sister, aunts, and uncles to let them know. They need to have some time to get over the shock before they see Mom again. They all know she hasn't felt good and wonder what is wrong but I don't think anyone knows how bad it actually is.
Even my sister, who is as close to Mom as I am doesn't know how bad it is. She lives further away from Mom than I so she doesn't see her quite as often. The last time she saw Mom was at Easter when Mom looked good but couldn't use her arm. Now she's not walking well, has little energy, and tires easily. Mom is physically exhausted and needed some rest.

My heart is breaking and I want to stay with them forever. I know they need some time to themselves to process everything we've just heard, so I decide to go home. As difficult as it is I go ahead and tell them I am going to go home and will be back in a few days.

I sadly tell Mom to get some rest and try not to worry too much and that I love her.

As I'm driving home I cry and wonder what will happen in the months to follow. How will I help care for Mom?

- When giving bad news practice empathy and compassion:
  - Be sensitive to the fact that the person you are informing may be so stunned that they misinterpret, completely deny, or even refuse to hear.
  - Be sensitive to their emotions: disbelief, shock, numbness, and anger are all part of the process.
  - Let them know that you care and are as concerned as they are. Try to refrain from letting your emotions take over and make the situation more tragic.
  - Answer any questions that they may have but try not to go into too many details during this initial discussion, especially if they are in denial.
  - Be realistic and don't make the situation worse by offering unrealistic statements that offer false hope.

- o Try to refrain from making statements such as "it hurts me as much as it does you." These statements don't offer much sympathy because you really don't know how they feel. What does help is for you to be a sounding board and listener, rather than a problem solver.
- o Family and friends will ask many questions, especially if you are taking the lead in the care. Be honest but not hurtful.

One of my friends told me that it's alright to cry and I do softly while talking to my family. I try very hard to remain calm while discussing what has happened. Everyone is so sad and it breaks my heart.

I know the family thinks I'm so strong but deep down my heart is dying a little more as each minute passes. I know I have to be the strong one to help Mom and Dad through this process and I pray for the strength I need to stay strong.

Chapter 5

Informing the Family

I call my youngest brother (Vegas) and he is shocked and horrified! He adores our parents and will do anything for them. He asks what he can do to help and I tell him the best thing would be to visit Mom. He said that he would get home as soon as possible. We talk and cry quietly and he tells me to let Mom know that he loves her.

He's in the process of buying a house so needs to take care of those details before traveling. He has talked about having my brother move in with him when Mom and Dad sell the house. Now that Mom is ill my brother that lives with them will eventually move in with my Vegas brother. So the timing was right for my Vegas brother to buy a house. He's so sad and asked me to look for flights within the next few months for him. "Of course I will," I say sadly.

I then call my oldest brother (California) and he is just as shocked and stunned. He doesn't see our parents very often and had no idea Mom was this ill. I tell him that he has to do whatever he can to visit this year. He asked me how long Mom had to live and I tell him honestly that we really don't know. We cry together softly as our hearts break.

I save the most difficult call for last, my sister. She's forty-seven but will always be my baby sister. I take some time for myself before calling her because I know how sad it will be. When I give her the news she cries and cries, and can't stop crying. We cry together for awhile and she keeps saying she can't believe it's that bad.

She says over and over, "Oh San, what are we going to do?" She's called me San for as long as I can remember. I calm myself down and tell her that we will do whatever we can to help Mom get through this. She said she is going to help as much as she can and says that she will do whatever we need her to do. It's very difficult to end the call with her because we are both so sad. I told her to call me anytime she needed to talk.

I call my Mom's sister the next day. She cries and wants me to know that she doesn't want to lose her only sister. Their other sister passed away last year and she is heartbroken. My aunt and uncle recently bought a place near my Mom and Dad and they all planned to have fun during their retirement. Now that dream is gone.

My Dad's sister calls me the next day crying.

Oh My Gosh, how am I going to do this? I quietly pray to God and ask him to help me through these horrible months to come and to give me the strength to help my family.

My Dad's sister is so upset and sad. She has not been healthy and will not be able to make a two hour trip to see Mom. We talk through it and I explain what has happened. I don't know how I'm doing this. Everyone is crying when I talk to them and I'm somehow able to explain the situation.

The only answer is that God is walking me through every waking moment.

I can't believe this is happening to our family. I've heard of tragic things happening to friends and diseases hitting so many families but I could never imagine how difficult it was. Things like this just don't happen to our family. I don't know how I'm going to do this. I have to remain strong for Mom and Dad. I feel like I'm' going to die a little day by day. Someone help me, help me, help me, deal with this tragedy.

Chapter 6

The First Month after the Diagnosis

July 2010:

I'm at Mom and Dad's once or twice a week. Mom feels better when people are visiting and she says it gives her energy and keeps her spirit's high. Mom's brothers and sister have visited as well as friends and neighbors. My sister and her family were here for the weekend and they cleaned carpets and brought all of the clothing up from the basement. The clothes are on racks in the garage and we'll go through them to decide what they need and what they can get rid of.

Everyone brings food so Dad doesn't always have to cook. They've had so much food and Mom and Dad are enjoying it well! One of the signs of progression is not eating well so it makes me happy that Mom is eating these days.

Mom is still able to walk slowly to the dining room table to eat. We purchase a chair disc that sits on top of the seat and spins on the chair when Mom moves her feet. This helps her sit on the chair and move easily from one side to the other without having to actually move her body.

Mom takes a nap while dinner is being cleaned up. After her nap I ask if she wants to clean out her closet. She said, "Yes, we should go ahead and get all these clothes cleaned out."

I start working on the closet while she sits on the bed. I take everything out. We will decide one by one what items she will keep in the closet. We are having fun as we go through the clothes and talk about different places we've been when she was wearing different outfits. She hesitates on many items and I say, "You haven't worn this for a year, do you really think you will wear it again?" We laugh and she says to get rid of it!

I'm secretly thinking that she probably won't wear most of what we keep. I don't want to discourage her by getting rid of too many things. When everything was put back together we ended up having eight boxes of clothes, purses, and shoes that we will give away or donate to the church.

My Dad talks to my cousin a few days later and she's able to take everything. She will keep some things, give some to her friends, and then donate the remaining items to the church.

Dad takes Mom to the casino whenever she's feeling up to it. She's very slow and tires easily but they do like to get out of the house while they still can. Spending a couple hundred dollars is nothing compared to the companionship and fun they have.

Mom's back and legs are getting weaker and she's having some difficulty walking around. Dad decided to go ahead and get her a wheelchair and says Mom really likes it. It's a small one that moves around the house easily. Actually it's so much easier on him since he has a bad back. It helps keep him stable while he's moving her around the house and out to the porch. I didn't think she would want one but she seems fine with it. I'm glad I had her use one at the doctor's office. It helped her realize how much physical energy she saves by not walking around the house.

Mom is already on Medicare because of her age. They pay some of the rental of the wheelchair. Dad's secondary insurance pays some and he ends up owing only $3.00 per month.

- **Get a Wheelchair as soon as possible. There are so many types of wheelchairs to choose from. Work with Medicare and your insurance company to determine which one will be covered by insurance. You can normally rent one and upgrade to a different one within a year. If you've contacted Hospice they may get the wheelchair for you. If you haven't contacted Hospice DO IT NOW!**

When I'm at the house I tell Mom to rest often because she is so tired all the time. Things certainly have changed. Mom used to go, go, go, and now she's lucky to get dressed for the day.

Our lives will never be the same.

I feel so good when I'm at Mom's but wonder how long I can do this. I ask Dad about moving in with us and selling the house. He does not want to sell the house until he absolutely has to, and I definitely understand. I tell him to please let me know when he's ready and we will do whatever we can to help.

Everything I read says to get things ready in advance before you have to. I will continue talking to them about moving in. I don't want to push it but feel that I may need to in the near future. It's so difficult to talk to Dad about what is happening. He is so sad and I cry too easy.

I'm so strong on the outside but can only take so much at a time. We've never really talked much about death and now we need to. I had their Health Care Power of Attorney and Living Will done before this happened, so that helps. I'm so thankful that I asked them about the legal papers a few years ago before anything happened.

"Please God just let her be free of pain"

I feel myself praying daily. I've always had faith and believe in God but haven't been openly religious. During these past few months I find myself wanting to go to church more often. I'm sure it's what is keeping me together and helping me get through the days. My daughter and I visited a new church last week and it felt so good. I know God hears me because he is walking me through this terrible time in my life. I don't expect miracles. I just ask that Mom to be free of pain. I also ask God to give me the strength I need to help my family.

My husband, how did I get so lucky? He says we will do whatever we need to do: build on to our house, buy a bigger house, move furniture around, whatever needs done. We are getting estimates to build on to the house in case my parent's do move in with us. I've also looked at houses to buy to see if there's anything we may want instead of building on. After looking at a few we decide that we really want to stay in our house. Mom and Dad are comfortable in our house and building on wouldn't be a bad thing. So we will probably build on while downsizing some of the furniture and make a few changes so that there is ample space for a wheelchair to get around.

One of my friends has helped her family with reorganizing a house to accommodate a wheelchair. She offers to come to our house to help decide what will need done. We go from room to room to review handicap options and talk about things that will help Mom.

- Make sure doorways are large enough for a wheelchair to move through easily
- Ramps to get in and out of the house
- Handicapped bathroom set-up
- Furniture that they can sit in for a long period of time
- Chairs and couch that are firm enough to get in and out of
- Trays, utensils, and bibs for eating
- Rugs need taken up so the wheelchair can move easily from room to room
- It's also a good idea to put plastic strips on doorways to protect the walls

I've decided to start talking to Mom about childhood and adult memories. My Mom and her sisters have talked quite often about their childhood and I wanted to hear more. They have so many funny stories and we would sit around the kitchen table and laugh and laugh. Especially the stories about walking a mile in two feet of snow with holes in their shoes! I think I even used that one with my daughters!

I knew there was so much more to hear. She's already told me about grandma but I want to hear more of her childhood, her romance with Dad, and when we were all little kids.

- Do this now! If you want to document childhood memories or any type of memory, do it now. I said I was going to do it and never actually got around to it. Time passed by so quickly. Also, if you want to go through old pictures or any type of memories, DO IT NOW! I didn't get a chance to go through all the pictures with Mom until it was too late. I was doing it by myself for the funeral memorial. We would have had so much fun looking at all those pictures and laughing at everything we've been through. I'm so sorry I didn't make this a priority.

After the funeral my Dad, my brother, and I went through a couple huge boxes Mom had in the basement. We laughed and laughed at all the great memories. We even found Moms senior report card! We sat for what seemed like hours pulling out different pieces of memories for all the siblings.

So do this now before it's too late!

I normally go to my parent's house on Wednesday and Thursday and then again on Saturday so I can help Dad as much as possible with the house and cooking. My daughter and I own our business and I only have to work about three days per week. This is the perfect situation right now as it gives me this precious time to spend with Mom.

I'm so thankful that I was able to retire early and start this business with my daughter. If I was still in the corporate life I would not have the time I need to be able to help them.

When I arrive in the afternoon some friends from the neighborhood are visiting and Mom looks happy. It is really amazing how many people are visiting and calling! I know Mom is truly loved and she seems really happy that so many friends and family members are around.

After they leave she is happy but tells me she really doesn't want anyone visiting anymore unless I'm there. She feels more comfortable when I'm there to help her. I'm able to see when she's getting tired or having trouble talking and can ask them to come back at another time when Mom is feeling up to it. Everyone certainly understands the situation.

I can't even imagine what Mom is thinking, *"Could this be my last month of life? Have I done everything I need to do? Will I be scared? Will God take care of me? Will it hurt? Will I cry? Will someone be with me? Will I be able to stay at home? Have I helped my kids as much as I could? Is there anything I need to tell them? Will they be happy? I will miss my family."*

I'm wondering how I'm going to talk to Mom about these things when I'm not sure what she wants or needs to say? We talk about the family all the time but how far do I dig into her thoughts and questions?

The one thing she thinks about often is my sister. My sister is very close to Mom and is having a difficult time accepting what is happening. Mom worries about her and I continue to reassure her that I will be here for my sister to lean on.

I want to start talking to Mom about these personal things but I'm so sad and it's difficult for me to start the conversations. If Mom brings them up I can discuss anything with her. The feeling is awful.

My daughter and I take the kids to see Mom and Dad on Wednesday. They love visiting with the kids. My grandson is eight and is understanding that great-gram's is sick and it's not a play day. He gives them a big hug and sits close to Dad for the day.

My other grandson is one year and they have fun watching him waddle through the house. It was a good day and Mom really enjoyed having them. But I can see the sadness in Mom's eyes when we leave. She knows there won't be many times like this left for her.

I go by myself on Friday to cook and clean and got so much done! Mom and Dad appreciate everything so much and I love helping them. They are wonderful people and parents and they both deserve to be helped as much as possible. I'm so thankful that my health is good and I'm able to help with anything they need.

Bless my dad! He has already converted the bathroom for handicap assistance and Mom loves it! I got her a soap dispenser that works from the motion of her hand and she's laughing because Dad and I keep making the soap come out every time we are near it. It's good to see Mom laughing.

A portable toilet works great over top of the regular toilet because she can hold herself up on the bars when she's sitting down. Dad also put bars on the wall across from the toilet that Mom can hold on to when she sitting down and getting back up. She wants to be able to use the restroom on her own for as long as possible.

Dad or I go into the bathroom with her to make sure she sits down without falling. We go back in when she's getting up to help her if she needs it. So far she seems to be getting up and down without much trouble. The bars in the shower give her stability and confidence when standing. She's happy that she can still take a shower on her own.

- Convert the bathroom as soon as possible with handicap bars and a large shower. Things are happening with us so quickly that we hardly have the time to stay ahead of the needs. A walk-in bathtub that has a seat would probably work well, unless they can't lift their feet to get in.
- A portable potty also works very well. You can put it over the seat of the regular toilet or use it as is. They can use the bars on the portable potty to help them sit down and get back up.
- A raised toilet seat is a must. It can be used alone or with the portable potty standing over top of it.

Mom and I begin the conversation about the funeral. I know we have to talk about this but my heart isn't ready. I'm thinking to myself that it doesn't matter what I can or can't do, I need to do this for Mom. She wants me to help her decide what to do. I'm thankful we had talked about funerals, being cremated, cemetery plans, life insurance, and all those things long before she got sick.

This was a good start and I'm so glad she starting the conversation as it was easier for me to bring certain things up. She begins by saying that she still hasn't decided if she wants to be cremated or buried. We talk about it for some time and share our views. This is horrible talking about what has to be done.

We have different views on the subject but I want her to do what she wants and not what my personal opinion or plans are. I tell her that this is her decision and she should do what she wants. She eventually decides that she wants to be buried and not cremated. She tells me that she doesn't want the casket open at the funeral and I don't understand why.

She says that she doesn't want anyone seeing her looking like this. I tell her she will always be beautiful and ask her if she's sure because people won't care what she looks like. They love her want to pay their respects.

I cry a little and remember what a good friend of mine recently told me. It's ok for us to see each other cry. My friend took care of her parents and it felt good to cry together. What good advice she gave! We wipe our tears and move forward with our discussion. I think it actually helps us both get through this ordeal.

- **Make sure there is a Power of Attorney on file, a Will, a Health Care Power of Attorney and a Living Will. Hospice will ask about all these documents. They all need signed and notarized.**
- **If you haven't done so, notify Hospice now.**

Dad is talking about getting a bigger van in case he needs to get a wheelchair lift. I'm thinking he doesn't need to do that just yet but it's good that he's thinking ahead.

Mom and I are talking about cleaning out some of the things in her bedroom and she said she wants to give my niece one of her jewelry boxes. We talk about her jewelry and she tells me that she wants me to have one of her diamond rings. It's the one I've always loved! It has five diamonds for all five of us kids and she wants me to have it! I'm so thrilled, honored, and sad all at the same time.

She said she wants the girls to go through her jewelry to make sure everyone gets something. She doesn't have a lot of expensive jewelry, just sentimental. She said that she gave my sister one of her other diamond rings and that all the girls should get something nice. I agree and know that my daughters will be thrilled to get some of their grams jewelry.

It seems so unreal to be discussing what everyone should get when Mom is no longer here. I know it needs done but it's so sad. My heart breaks more every day.

I'm so blessed to have so much love and concern from my family, friends and acquaintances. There is an ALS walk coming up and my daughter and I decided that we should participate this year. We started recruiting family members and friends to walk with us.

I told Mom about it and she's even thinking of allowing us to walk her in the wheelchair. That would be so awesome! I know Mom and she worries so much about what she looks like that I secretly know she will never join us.

We started our plans and 'Team Gearhart' was formed in honor of Mom. We decided to use 'walk to defeat ALS' with a rainbow on the T-Shirts. The rainbow represents the fact that ALS can affect any life, any size, any color, and age. It's very touching and exciting to see how many people are going to contribute to the cause in honor of our Mom.

My girlfriend from high school is driving three hours to join the walk with her husband, my husband's friend is coming with his wife, his daughter's family and their dog, my sister and her family, my daughter and her family, and a few others are thinking about it. I know my heart will go out to the thousands of people joining the walk because they will all be there for the same reason.

Chapter 7

The Second Month after the Diagnosis

August 2010:

My sister and I met at Moms this weekend and I think this is the first time we have been together without our husband's in 20 years! It was nice and felt like we were kids again.

Mom is walking slower and feeling much weaker. I ask her if she's using her wheelchair much and she says some, but likes to walk if she can. She knows I worry about her falling and says she's very careful when she walks.

We talk quite a bit now about how things are and what will happen. She started reading some material I gave her about the disease and what to expect but she said it just depressed her and she couldn't really read much of it. She wants me to explain things to her as we go along.

It feels so weird that we have now gotten to the point that we can talk about the future and death. As hard as it is I'm so thankful that Mom is able to talk about it. I really think I'm the only one she can talk to and it makes her feel good that I will do whatever she needs or wants.

Mom wants to talk about what is happening and what to expect next. I explain to her that her left arm has lost all muscle function and that her right one will probably lose muscle function next. Her shoulder has been sore since the arm started to lose function and she doesn't know why.
I explained that the information I read says that the arm hangs down when it loses function and sometimes dislocates itself. I tell her a sling might help but she doesn't want to use that. She says her arm doesn't hurt if she keeps it resting on her lap.

I also told her that once her legs get much weaker she will need to use her wheelchair full time. She worries about not being able to use her legs and I explain that Dad and I will be able to help her bathe and move around the house.

I explain that, hopefully, the last muscle to lose function will be her mouth, throat and breathing muscles. Once they lose function, she won't be able to eat and then her breathing muscles will stop. I tell her that her mind and bowels should always stay normal and she will be aware of what is happening.

She is sad but thanks me for helping her understand what is happening. I hug her often these days and tell her I love her. She knows it but needs as much comfort as we can give at this time in her life.

We had previously talked about a ventilator and feeding tube and Mom told me she doesn't want either one. She tells me again today and I told her I will get all the legal papers out because I want to make sure we have everything signed and notarized. I'm concerned about the ventilator and feeding tube.

I explain to her that my concern is, If her mind is alert and I tell my siblings that Mom doesn't want the intervention they may get upset and blame me. Mom said, "They won't," and I told her, "I don't think they will blame me but it would be easier if everything is in writing. That way, there's no question and Dad will even understand." I make a mental note to make sure I talk to Dad about this to see if Mom has discussed it with him also

- **With ALS the mind normally stays sharp for the duration of the disease.**

Mom tells me that no one can understand the feeling. Her legs are getting heavy and she says they get harder and harder to pick up. They don't hurt but just feel heavy. Her arm is the same way. The only thing that hurts every now and then is her shoulder.

She asks, *"Do you have any idea of how fast it will progress?"* I honestly say, *"I really don't know, the doctor told us it could be six months or six years."* I told her, *"It would really be nice if you just stayed this way for many years."* But, she says, *"No it will go faster, I can tell."* I tell her *"I hope not Mom, but we will deal with it the best we can and I'll do everything I can to help you."* Our eyes are showing the sadness in both of us. She always thanks me for helping her and Dad and that she appreciates everything I do. I'm so sad that I'm losing my Mom and she is just as sad that she is in the last phase of her life. She loves being around her family and knows how much we will miss her. I feel that this disease is hitting her hard and fast and really don't think she will be with us another year.

It doesn't seem real to me. I feel like I'm a robot. I'm caring for my Mom and helping Dad as much as possible but I can't get it around my mind that I'm really losing my Mom.

How do people do this?

Dad decided to buy a used conversion van. He wants to make sure there is room for a wheelchair lift. He's handling things pretty well; even though I know his heart is breaking more and more every day. I'm not sure how he will handle this once Mom is gone.

He keeps asking Mom if she wants to go for a ride and she always says that she really doesn't want to go anywhere. I feel bad for him as he is trying everything he can do to help Mom get around. He thinks she will feel better if she takes a ride in the van every now and then.

She just doesn't want to leave the house. I think she is terrified that she may get hurt and Dad won't be able to help her. I tell her that I will go with them anywhere she wants to go and she still says that she would like to stay home for now, maybe later.

My sister and I clean the house and pick up some of the throw rugs. Mom doesn't need to be tripping on those darn rugs. She loves her throw rugs! Mom is laughing quite a bit during the weekend and it sounds nice. She starts laughing then can't get up from a chair or do anything.

We are having fun and we're so close these days. I just love my parent's. I pray daily that Mom doesn't have any pain with this disease. She is such a sweet person and this doesn't seem fair.

Mom is still smoking. At this point she figures, "Why not? I always liked smoking and thought cancer would kill me." My sister and I told her she might have to quit if she can't light her cigarette or hold it. We have never smoked and she laughed at the thought of us lighting her cigarette or holding it.

We know inside that we would do anything to help her. We all laugh about it and told her we would have Dad put something together that goes around her head to hold her cigarettes! She just laughs and laughs!

That evening we sit at the table a play a dice game called LCR, Mom loves it and we play for nickels and quarters and laugh for an hour or so. Mom can only use one arm and hand but she's doing really well. This is what we will miss, having fun with our Mom.

My sister and I sleep together that night. We talk and cry quietly about what is happening. We can't believe what we are going through but will do whatever we can to help. My sister says she doesn't know what she will do without Mom.

She is so heartbroken and can't accept what is happening. I hug her and tell her that I will always be here for her and we will get through this together. She always says that I'm the strong one. Deep down I'm heartbroken as much as she is but I try to remain as strong and calm as I can.

I'm so sad tonight.

"Dear Lord, please watch over my parents. My mom is so weak. Please help her through this without pain. My Dad is fighting his own battles with a bad leg and back, but he continues to help with everything. Please continue to give him the strength he needs to stay strong. I am so blessed that you are giving me the strength I need. Amen."

I'm sure it wasn't the first time and it won't be the last time that my sister and I cried softly as we fell asleep.

The remaining weekend went along nice. We played LCR again the following evening. Mom loves that game! We play for nickels and laugh for an hour. This is what we will miss, having fun with our Mom. I see that Mom is getting tired so I suggest that we watch a movie, knowing Mom will rest.

My sister and I sadly and slowly get ready to leave the next day. It breaks our hear to leave Mom and Dad. We know how sad they are and we hug them and then give each other a much needed bear hug before getting in our cars to go in different directions. We will always cherish this time with Mom.

The following weekend my Mom's sister and husband came over to play cards. They get together every few weeks and I'm so glad she's able to still do this for now. I got Mom a card holder to hold her cards since she isn't able to use her right arm. She's a little slower but it's working pretty well. Mom loves being able to play cards for now and I love to see her laugh and have fun.

Mom is walking so slow and unstable these days and I'm worried about her falling. She holds on to the walls or anything that she's near. She says she's very careful but I can see that she's having trouble walking. I told her she might need to get around in the wheelchair so she doesn't fall. She is using a cane and doesn't want to use the wheelchair unless she absolutely needs to. I know she will need to use it very soon though.

Her legs are so heavy and she can hardly pick her feet up off the floor to walk. She said it feels like her feet are bricks and that's exactly what it looks like when she walks. It's so painful watching her try to get around or do things.

She is still laughing often but I can tell she hates what is happening to her. She tells me, "I think the disease is progressing quickly and my right arm is starting to get weak. What will happen when I can't do anything with my right arm?" I say sadly, "We will do whatever needs done. We can feed you, dress you, help with bathing, or anything else." She says, "I hate that you have to do everything for me. But I'm so glad you're here." "I'm so happy I'm able to do this for you and I wouldn't want it any other way. I love you mom."

We sit quietly and think about the future.

Chapter 8

The Third Month after the Diagnosis

September 2010:

The disease is progressing quickly. I can't believe how fast this is taking over my Mom's body. She is walking very carefully and slowly these days. She uses a cane and holds on to the wall or whatever she is near when she walks. Her legs are getting weaker and weaker. She doesn't want to use the wheelchair all the time but I think she really needs to.

When I get to their house Dad tells me that Mom fell the other day but didn't get hurt. My brother that lives with them was able to help Dad get her up on the chair. I see the bruises on her arm and leg and ask her if she feels alright. She tells me she didn't get hurt but it scared her.

I can only imagine how frustrating this is for her. I told her how worried I am that she fell and that she really needs to use the wheelchair. She smiles in a childlike way and says she will use the wheelchair more. I try to make light of it and act like her mother when I say "If you fall again you know you will need to move in with us." She laughs and says that she knows. Sometimes it's just easier to make light of the subject and smile or laugh a little.

Dad bought Mom a reclining chair with an automatic lift in it. She absolutely loves it! She said it's so easy to get up and down. This is just what she needed so that she doesn't have to use so much energy to get up or sit down. Dad said she thinks she's Queen of the house with her new chair!

It kills me to see that she has to use this chair but I'm happy that she doesn't need to use so much energy sitting down and getting up. She said it's comfortable and she doesn't mind sitting in it for a few hours at a time.

The lift chair was perfect timing. Mom's bowels are moving more often these days and she has to get up and down every hour or so. Her stomach isn't upset and she says she isn't sick. Food just doesn't stay in her system very long. It could be her medicine or just the changes in her body and health but we don't want her getting dehydrated, so Dad will call the doctor if it continues.

Someone has to help Mom get in and out of the lift chair so that she doesn't fall. She uses the automatic control and lifts herself up and will stand for a little while to get stable. We hold on to her body while she turns slowly to sit in the wheelchair. She's very unstable now and uses tiny, tiny steps to move herself around.

I started looking on-line for medical supplies that could help her with any activity. I saw this large round disc that could be used to stand on while moving from one seat to another. I thought this would be great and purchased it immediately. It seemed very easy but Mom was worried that she would fall. It was worth a try but she was too nervous and frightened to try it. So we continue helping her move from bed to wheelchair to lift chair, and back. We will try anything to make things easier on her.

A Reclining lift chair is worth every penny. Medicare and secondary insurance may pay for some of it. If not, it's worth the cost. This helps them get up and down without using much energy. Mom said it's comfortable and she can sit in it for quite a long time. It looks like a normal reclining chair that you would use in your living room.

- Use a blanket or sheet to protect the chair if they have any type of bowel problem.
- We also tried different pillows under her and between her arms to keep her comfortable when she sits for a long period of time.
- We put a very small pillow under the arm that has no muscle so that she can keep it rested and not have to hold it up. Her arm is bent at the elbow and a small pillow helps keep it comfortable.

The September birthdays are such a terrific tradition for our family. I'm so sad that this will probably be the last one with my Mom. The birthdays include Mom, my brother, my daughter, two nieces, my granddaughter, and my grandson. My daughter and her family were able to fly in from Phoenix for the celebration this year. We meet at Mom's house over Labor Day weekend and Dad makes sure he orders Mom's favorite white cake with white icing.

I'm both sad and happy over the weekend. I love having the family together with the kids playing and laughing. But I'm sad to know that this may be our last birthday tradition with Mom at the center. What will we do when Mom is gone?

We will definitely carry on the tradition in her name. We had so much fun and Mom really enjoyed herself. She was weak but she held up all day with the exception of one small nap. She laughed and loved watching the grandkids and great grandkids play out in the yard and ride around on their golf cart.

The only real problem she had was losing her breath every now and then. She's starting to have problems if there is any kind of smell in the air. I forgot to tell the girls to not wear perfume and the smell would sometimes cause her to have breathing problems when they hugged her. Of course they want to hug her!

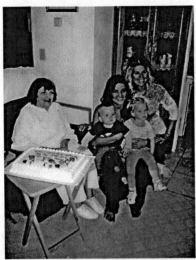

Some of the September birthdays, still smiling!

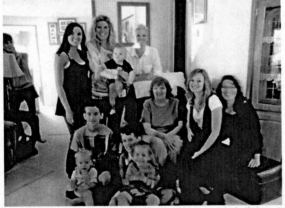

Mom with a portion of her grandchildren and great grandchildren, at her 76th birthday party. All smiles! Mom normally wears her gown and robe during the day but today was special. She wanted to wear pants and a nice top when everyone got there. I combed her hair, put on some make-up and chose something simple to wear. She looked good and seemed happy.

Mom wanted to go outside and she told me that she didn't want everyone coming on the porch with us.   The porch is huge and she just wanted to sit outside with my sister and me. We told her everyone was busy riding the golf cart and playing with the kids and it would be ok.

We got her outside in her wheelchair and don't you know it, everyone ended up on the porch! It's obvious that everyone wanted to be around Mom as much as possible. The only thing we could do was laugh with Mom!

My Dad, brother-in-law and husband were discussing building a ramp to the house. Mom needs to use her wheelchair most of the time now and won't be able to walk down the steps to the car. These guys will have the ramp figured out and built in no time! I would like them to wait because I wanted to talk to Dad more about staying with us.

I figured I will give up asking them to move in and just ask them to stay with us for awhile. That way he can keep the house and my brother can take care of it while they are at our house. Dad can also go to the house every week or so to check on my brother and the house. Mom's health is deteriorating so fast that I really hate for Dad to make too many structural changes.

I knew it would be sad when everyone left for the day and I could tell it was on their minds. We had a wonderful time watching everyone open their birthday gifts, especially the funny hats that were given out for the kids to wear. We didn't want that to end but it was time for everyone to begin thinking about leaving. They were all wondering if they would ever see their grams again or if this was going to be the last time they saw her alive.

As we took those final pictures outside everyone had tears in their eyes and it broke my heart. Everyone is trying to be strong but their hearts are all breaking. They hug Mom and Dad and tell them that they love them.

I look at my daughter and I know she is worried about seeing her grams again because she lives across the country. Her faith is strong and she knows she will see her grams in heaven but it's still so sad. It takes all I have to maintain my composure while everyone was saying goodbye.

We knew this would probably be the last big birthday celebration with Mom and it was agonizing thinking of everyone's broken heart. We all hugged with sad tears in our eyes and I wanted to scream in agony.

Why does it have to be like this? It's not fair.

When we get home everyone feels sad and exhausted. My daughter and her family, from Phoenix, were staying with us for the week. I normally play and laugh with the kids and help as much as I can. This week is different. I don't have the energy and my mind is always on Mom. When my daughter and I were alone in the bedroom I knew it was time to have a discussion about how I was feeling.

 I apologized for not treating them the way I normally do. I said that I was really sorry for not having fun and watching the kids like I should be. She tells me that she is worried about me and hopes I'm taking care of my health. She sees the difference in me when I'm at Moms compared to when I'm home worrying about Mom. She said she could see the stress lift from me when I'm with my Mom. She also sees that all I do is worry when I'm not with Mom.

She's right. Every waking moment I am consumed with thoughts of Mom. I wonder if I'm doing enough to help them, I wonder if she's feeling ok when I'm not around, I wonder if Dad is able to help Mom, and I wonder how soon I can get back out to their house.

My daughter says that she understands what I'm going through and tells me to take care of myself. We cry softly about what we are going through. I tell her this may be her in twenty years, taking care of me. She tells me she doesn't know how I'm doing it but so glad that I'm able to care for her grams. She tells me she can't stand to see me this sad but knows how much I love my Mom, just as she loves me. We needed this talk and hug each other tightly.

My husband and I were talking about the weekend with the family at Moms. I told him that it was good to see him sitting and talking with Mom. I could hear her telling him how she felt when it first started and that she couldn't understand why she was so tired. He said that she wanted to keep talking about her condition, so he let her talk as much as she wanted. He said it seemed like she wanted someone to talk to.

My husband is a great listener and very comforting. I'm sure he made her feel comfortable enough to talk about what was happening to her. He told me he couldn't believe how fast her health is deteriorating. He saw her about a month ago and the changes astonished him.

Mom talks to me quite a bit about her condition and I felt good that she could talk to him about it.

The following week I make sure to come over on September 8th to celebrate Mom's 76th birthday. Happy Birthday Mom, I love you with all my heart! It's really difficult to figure out what to get Mom this year. She doesn't really need anything and she's not getting out much.

I've been bringing things to the house as she needs them so there isn't anything she wants or needs. I did go ahead and get her a new blouse and jacket to wear if she does get out of the house. She loved it and said she hoped she could wear it sometime soon. We both secretly knew that she would probably never wear it. I've also been buying her new nightgowns and robes since that is really all she is wearing during the day.

- **Silk nightgowns are the easiest for her to wear as they will slide with her rather than pull against her when she moves at night. She's also wearing the silk nightgowns during the day with a cotton robe. It's easier for her to wear the nightgowns and robes. She can't move around very well in pants and shirts, and going to the bathroom is much easier.**
- **Once Hospice is involved they will bring hospital gowns to wear.**

I manage to come every week at one time or another and THANK GOODNESS I was here tonight. Mom's legs were really feeling heavy and she is having a difficult time walking at all. She said they get heavier at night and her legs and feet are beginning to swell quite a bit. I'm sure it's because she doesn't exercise them much and she's retaining water.

Mom was getting up from her lift chair which lifts her up to a standing position. She was turning a little to sit in her wheelchair and lost her footing and fell.

OH MY GOSH, this can't be happening, this is horrible, I can't catch her, and someone help me.

 I couldn't catch her because I was on the other side of the wheelchair holding it for her to sit in. Dad was sitting in a chair on the other side of the room. She's been getting up with us standing with the wheelchair so we thought she would be fine. She lost her balance and couldn't hold on to anything because her arms don't have any strength in them. I was so worried she hurt herself. Thank goodness she fell slowly on the carpet and didn't hit her head or anything.

She moaned and started crying immediately and I jumped on the floor to help her move to one side. She was crying and I wanted to make sure her shoulder wasn't injured. I was holding her in my arms on the floor and we were both crying.

"How can I help her? She is so sad, terrified, and scared. My heart is breaking, please help me help her."

This is so sad and I just don't know how I'm going to do it. Her teeth fell out of her mouth. I could see in her eyes that she was terrified. She looked like a little child that had fallen and couldn't move. Dad and I sat with her on the floor as we calmed her down. She was crying, "You won't be able to move me, how are you going to get me up? You can't do it." She was so scared but, thank goodness, wasn't hurt.

I told her I would lift her to the couch and she said that there isn't any way I could lift her. I really thought I would be able to and put my arms under her arms and tried to pull her up. I wasn't even thinking she would be dead weight, but she was and I couldn't even budge her. My dad thought about putting a blanket under her, pulling her over to the couch, and lifting her up on the couch with the blanket under her.

My brother that lives with them was downstairs. He didn't hear what was going on so I called for him to come and help us. She was crying and kept saying, "*You can't pick me up. How will I get up? You can't do it. What are we going to do? What will happen?*" I kept hugging her and telling her that we would figure it out. At least she wasn't hurt.

We rolled her to one side and put the blanket under her. Then rolled her to the other side and pulled the blanket out so that she was completely on the full blanket. We pulled the blanket slowly over the floor to the couch. She was crying sadly. My brother, Dad and I each took a corner of the blanket and pulled her up on the couch. It worked! We were all happy that we got her on the couch.

Mom was so upset and just kept crying. I'm hugging her and thinking to myself that I can't do this. I will never forget the look in her eyes when she was on the floor. How much harder is this going to get before it gets any better? This is breaking our hearts.

Mom has never cried as much as she has in the past few months. I feel so sorry for her. She hates that she can't do anything. I sat on the couch with her while hugging her and rubbing her back and arms and telling her she would be alright.

She kept saying, "What am I going to do? Your dad can't lift me. I'm so glad you were here. What would we do if you weren't here? How are you going to lift me? What will we do? No one is strong enough."

I kept hugging her and rubbing her back and telling her that we will figure it out one way or the other. She finally settled down and said she was ready to go to bed. This took all the energy she had and she was physically and emotionally exhausted. We get her to the bedroom in the wheelchair and Dad dresses her for bed. The next morning Dad said she was anxious all night and couldn't sleep. She is so worried about falling asleep and not being able to get back up, or not waking up at all.

- **Crying is typical with ALS. See information on Spastic Bulbar Palsy in the reference guide at the back of the book.**

One of my good girlfriends told me to start lifting weights to gain upper body strength and now I know why. My Dad definitely can't lift Mom by himself because he has a bad back and knee. I will need to do the best I can to help him. We can also think about getting a lift to help her in and out of bed if we need to.

- **There are several different kinds of lifts to move the patient from bed to wheelchair and back**
- **If Hospice is involved they may be able to recommend a lift or get one through their program**

Mom's breathing has started giving her problems. When Mom smells anything like cleaner, lotion, perfume, powder, or anything with a scent she starts shallow breathing and can hardly talk. She will ask us to turn the air on, turn it off, open or shut the window, put the fan on or off, and just about anything to help give her air. Part of the problem is that she is still smoking. Part of it is anxiety and she's worried she won't be able to breathe. This has been going on for a few weeks now so Dad called the doctor to see what he could do to help Mom.

Her Doctor prescribed an inhaler and Dad went to pick it up. It's similar to what people use to help them breath better if they have asthma. Mom hasn't been sleeping well and Dad is hoping this helps relieve a little anxiety. She has anxiety about not being able to breathe and is afraid she won't be able to prop herself up. Dad said he was going to have her do the inhaler when she goes to bed tonight, hoping that will help her sleep.

- An Inhaler may help if the patient is having any trouble breathing. Do this as soon as the patient seems to be having any trouble breathing or gets short of breath when there is a smell in the room. An inhaler will help for the time being. At a later date you may need to get a breathing treatment machine called a Nebulizer, or Oxygen.

Mom and I talked about grandma tonight. When things happen to her she talks about similar things that happened to grandma. Grandma lived with Mom and Dad for a few years before she passed away. She had a heart condition and got weaker and weaker until her heart gave out. Mom said that grandma used to sleep sitting up because she was worried about lying down and not being able to get back up.

Mom told me all about grandma and her last days. She has told me the story many times but I think it helps her when she talks about Grandma. I think she has some comfort in knowing she will see her Mom and Sister in heaven sometime soon. I know that's what Mom is worried about tonight. She was thinking about sleeping in her lift chair but Dad was able to talk her into going to bed with him.

We got Mom a large wedge pillow to lie on when she's in bed, hoping that it will help her breathe better and have less anxiety. The pillow helps keep her upper body at a 30% angle so that she isn't laying flat on the bed. She said it helped a little but she doesn't really like it. We will need to get a hospital bed soon or some kind of bed that automatically inclines so that she can sleep with her upper body at an incline.

When they get up the next morning, Dad says that Mom had a difficult night because she has too much anxiety. He sleeps next to her to help keep her calmer but it doesn't seem to be working very well these days. We need to talk to the doctor about some anxiety medicine and think about getting an automatic bed or hospital bed very soon. I begin researching automatic beds on the internet so that we can understand what options there are.

Mom tells me she just can't rest and that she sleeps a little while and then wakes up. I tell her that I think she needs to use the wedge pillow so that she's not laying flat on the bed and that we are looking into an automatic bed for her. She's frustrated because she can't sleep at night. She sleeps well during the day in her recliner but I think that's because she is sitting up and she knows that we are awake to keep an eye on her.

When we were sitting outside tonight I talked to Mom quite a bit about moving in with us. She hates to do that because she doesn't want to burden us. I told her they didn't have to sell the house and that they could just come and stay with us for awhile so we can help more. My brother already lives with them so he can stay at the house and Dad can go to the house every week to see how things are. That way she would have my Dad, me, my husband, my daughter, and her husband near her.

My daughter only lives ten minutes from us so they are close enough to come to the house if we're not home. I told her I would feel so much better and it would be easier for all of us. I would be with her every day and wouldn't need to drive over an hour to get to them once a week for a day or so. She kept saying, "*I don't know what to do. I won't get any better and will need constant care.*"

I try to reassure her that we will take care of her and she doesn't need to worry. I tell her that Dad and I will continue caring for her full time and will only need the others to help once in awhile. She knows Dad can't do this alone and keeps saying that she was so glad I was here when she fell.

Mom needs to be around me more. I know it and she knows it. For some reason she thinks I can handle everything and that I will know what to do if anything happens. So far, I've been strong and have been able to help with everything but who knows what will happen next.

"Please God, just give me the strength to continue being strong for them."

My California brother called tonight to talk to Mom and she only talked for a few minutes before her energy gave out. She was having trouble talking and breathing. She said it gets worse when she is anxious or excited and both happen when any of my siblings call. She misses her children and doesn't see them enough.

I saw that she was having trouble so I took the phone and talked to my brother and he just kept saying, "Oh no, Oh no." I don't think he thought it was as bad as it is and he doesn't realize what ALS is. I explained some of the symptoms of ALS and asked him to look at some of the ALS websites so that he could learn a little more about the disease and what Mom is going through.

I was very serious when I said to him, "Please try to get home as soon as you can to visit with Mom, she needs to see you while she's still able to talk and visit. She is so sad and wants to see you and our other brother from Vegas." Mom told me that she really hopes both my brothers get home before her health deteriorates too much. He said he's been working so much overtime and it's been hard for him to schedule a trip, but will try as soon as possible.

My Vegas brother called her last week and Mom had to give the phone to Dad because she couldn't talk. She started crying and was so upset and I know my brother didn't know what to do. He called me the next day to talk about it. He is so upset and I can only imagine how he feels. If I wasn't near Mom I would feel terrible not being able to see her and care for her. He told me he wanted to come home as soon as he could and asked me to find him an airline ticket. I told him I would see what I could find for him.

My niece called to talk to Mom and I told Mom not to tell her about the fall. We didn't need my sister and niece any more upset then they already are. My sister falls apart when something happens to Mom and then Mom starts crying. She can hardly talk about it and walks away when Mom and I start talking about anything to do with the future or how Mom is progressing. They talked for just a few minutes before Mom was struggling to talk. Mom looked at me as if to tell me to take the phone. She handed me the phone and I talked to my niece for awhile and told her that I hoped to see her soon.

My niece has the same birthday as Mom and they share a very special bond. She's 18 and this is the first time someone in the family has been ill. She's not quite sure how to handle it because her Mom is so sad and I think to myself that I will do what I can to comfort her.

Mom, Dad and I go to bed and I'm sitting here crying as I type this. I can hardly see the computer because of all the tears. My heart is aching and I've cried more in the past few months then I have in a year. I try not to cry around Mom or Dad during the day but need the release at night as I type my journal while resting in bed.

I accept what's happening and I'm strong for them but my heart breaks more and more every day. Writing this journal is very therapeutic for me but I'm still heartbroken and can't imagine what our lives with be like without Mom.

"Dear Lord, please give us the strength to get through this. Thank you for everyday you give us on earth and I pray that you help Mom get through this horrible disease without much pain. Amen"

Mom is amazed at all the visitors she's had over the last few months. She loves visiting but it's getting more and more difficult for her to talk for a very long time. The inhaler is helping her breath a little easier and it seems to help keep her calmer and be less anxious about breathing. She's using the inhaler more often during the day now to help with her breathing.

I'm so glad it's getting a little cooler outside with some air blowing around. She loves to go outside and hasn't been able to very much because it's been so hot with no air moving around. Since her fall she's decided to start using the wheelchair fulltime now to move from her bed to the reclining chair and back.

I can see her right arm and legs getting weaker and weaker. She shows me how her legs are getting weaker. She can hold her legs up when she's sitting down but can't pick them up when she's standing on them. It's so sad and I pray every day for the Lord to watch over her and keep her from pain.

- **Make sure you have a wheelchair available before the legs are too weak to walk. Sometimes it happens so fast that one day the legs seem fine but the next day the patient needs to use a wheelchair.**
- **Range of motion exercises are needed to keep the legs and arms from getting stiff.**

I was able to get my Vegas brother a flight the following week and he came home for two weeks. He hasn't seen Mom for a year. I talk about what is happening to Mom on the drive from Columbus to their home. I want him to understand what she is going through and that she can't walk or do very much for herself. He knows she can't talk very long since she had to hand the phone to my Dad when they were talking last week. She started crying because she couldn't breathe very well and my brother said it broke his heart.

When we arrive at Mom's he runs in the house and hugs her for about five minutes. He couldn't let her go and she was so happy to see him. It's so difficult because he lives so far away and they both know this could actually be the last time he sees her alive. We have a nice evening and he always has everyone laughing, which was no different this time.

He was very good with her and was able to ask some difficult questions and talk about the disease. It's better if they understand what is happening to her. He didn't know very much about the disease so our discussion helped him understand everything she was going through.

I take over when I'm at Mom's so that Dad can take a good break from everything and relax a little. I was helping Mom get from the wheelchair to her lift chair and my Dad says, "*Sandra, you should have been a nurse! You are so good with people.*" Mom agrees and I just chuckle and say, "*I'm not sure about that, I might not be as nice to someone else.*" They laughed and both of them say how much they appreciate everything I do to help them.

On the inside I'm thanking them for allowing me to care for Mom. It helps me understand what is happening and I feel so good knowing that she is well taken care of. I feel honored that they allow me to help with everything that needs completed for the next phase of their life. I can't imagine not taking over as caregiver and love being around them often.

I've always been a compassionate person but there is nothing like true compassion until you are a caregiver to someone you love.

I get ready to leave so that my brother can spend some quality time with Mom for the two weeks that he is home.

Sept 26, 2010:

Today was the Walk to Defeat ALS in Columbus, Ohio. We had a good group walk for my Mom and we were able to donate over $1,300 to the ALS Association! The company that made our T-shirts gave us half off the price; which was his donation to the cause. We had a great time! I had some anxiety about the walk and later figured it was because I would see such a large group of people supporting the same cause. I wanted to hug everyone and cry with them. I posted pictures on face book and had so many great comments from family and friends.

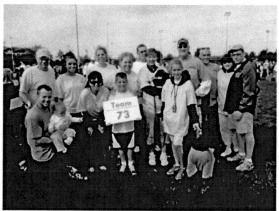

Family and Friends at the ALS Walk: 'Team Gearhart'

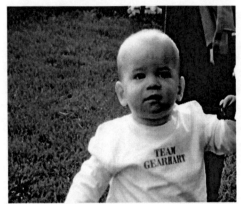

My grandson Justin

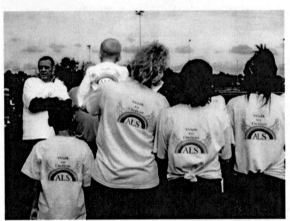

Our team shirts were a big hit!

Chapter 8

The Fourth Month after the Diagnosis

October 2010:

I can't believe how fast this disease is taking over my Mom's body. She doesn't talk very long now because her voice gives out. Any kind of smell takes her breath away and she has difficulty breathing: perfume, flowers, dust, laundry detergent, bath products, and cleaning supplies. We've changed to free and clear everything!

- **Once the patient starts having a difficult time being around any kind of smell, IMMEDIATELY switch to free and clear laundry detergent, house cleaning supplies, and bath products. When someone visits ask them to NOT wear perfume or any strong sprays.**

My Dad and Vegas brother talked Mom into getting out of the house for a ride to the Casino to play some slot machines. I can't believe they were able to talk her into it but I'm pretty sure she agreed because she knew my brother would be able to lift her if anything happened. Dad had my brother build a wooden step to sit on the ground that Mom could use to get into the van.

She was worried that she would fall but my brother wheeled her down the ramp that they built and was able to lift her into the van. He helped her out of the van into the wheelchair when they arrived and things worked out pretty well. They only stayed about an hour but it was good to get her out of the house. Dad was so happy that she was able to get out for awhile.

My Vegas brother left on October 5th, to go back home. My husband and I came over to the house to pick him up and take him to the airport. It was so sad and broke our hearts. Both Mom and my brother cried when he had to leave. They hugged and hugged and didn't want to let the other one go. We all know that it was because of the uncertainty of Mom's health.

We know the disease will take her life but we don't have any idea exactly how long she will have. He was so sad and crying when we drove away. There isn't anything you can do to help someone in a situation like this but listen and give them support.

My husband was driving and I sat in the back seat with tears streaming down my face. I always cry when I leave Mom and I felt so sad for my brother. He has to go back to Vegas and the next time he sees Mom will probably be at her funeral.

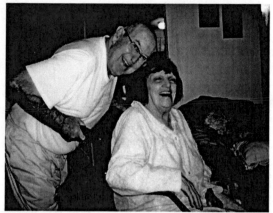
Mom and Dad 10/4/2010, still smiling

My Vegas brother took this picture. He sure has a way of making Mom laugh. He is definitely the comedian in the family and it was good to see her laughing so much. You can see how her left hand has formed into a 'claw'. Her eyes are also getting darker and darker these days.

Dad decided to get Mom a hospital bed and had it delivered this week. He called me and we talked about how much it should help her. He is hoping that it will help Mom sleep and be able to move around more comfortably. Her left shoulder is very painful so she needs to be careful when she moves. We're hoping that sleeping with her upper body at an incline she won't have as much anxiety about not being able to breathe.

When I get to Mom's the following week I asked her about the bed. She said she sleeps a couple hours then wakes up and can't get back to sleep. Most of the problem is anxiety and she's afraid she won't be able to move or wake up.

Dad had a doctor's appointment and he talked to the doctor about Mom. Her doctor ordered anxiety medicine and said it should help her relax and sleep better. Mom doesn't have any problem sleeping in her lift chair during the day, it's just at night. I think she's afraid that we won't hear her if she needs any help.

Dad and I talked to Mom about the medicine and explained that it would help ease her anxiety and help her sleep better. The doctor told Dad it was mainly for depression but we didn't want to talk to Mom about being depressed. Of course she's depressed. She has a disease that is going to take her life and she doesn't know how long she has to live.

She's worried about taking too much medicine and we keep telling her the medicine isn't going to hurt her. It will help her feel better and she should be able to sleep more than a few hours at a time. She finally said she would take the medicine. We are hoping it helps her. I know she's full of anxiety on the inside. I am amazed at how well she actually is on a daily basis but the night time is what bothers her so much.

I ask her if she wants to sleep in her chair tonight and she did. I sleep on the couch where I can keep an eye on her. I think one of her main worries is that Dad will be sleeping and won't be able to hear or help her if she has an anxiety attack or can't breathe.

She seemed to sleep pretty good in the chair but I knew I couldn't do that very often. The couch was very uncomfortable and I didn't get much rest at all which I will need if I'm going to stay healthy so that I can care for her.

Dad and I talked about her anxiety the next day and he said he was going to talk to her doctor about having a therapist or someone come and talk with her to help ease her anxiety. This is breaking my heart and I see how sad my Dad is and how his heart is also breaking.

He said he doesn't know what to do when she has an anxiety attack and starts crying during the night. He said he tries to comfort her but she starts crying and can't stop. I'm sure she cries more when she's with him and shares more of her fears about what is happening to her. Dad has been pretty strong but I'm not sure how much more he can take. I need to make sure I'm around them more so that Dad has someone to lean on.

Dad has been itching all over and he went to the doctor to figure out what it was. His doctor sent him to a dermatologist and they prescribed skin cream and anxiety medicine for him as well. They said this outbreak could be from all the stress he's going through. He tells us about it and Mom and I laughed about how everyone in the house will eventually be on depression or anxiety medicine.

I even had my yearly physical and told my doctor about Mom and she asked if I needed anything to help with my stress. I told her that I didn't need anything at that time but would let her know if I needed anything later. I don't want to take anything unless I absolutely need it and at this point I think I'm getting through it alright.

My daughter and I sold our business and it couldn't have happened at a better time. I've been spending a day or two at my parent's house and now I will be able to spend three to five days a week. My husband misses me but he understands how important it is for me to be with my parent's as much as possible. He helped care for his mother and understands the circumstances it brings.

My daughter and grandchildren also miss me. My nine year old grandson normally stays all night with me each week and isn't able to as much now. He knows I'm taking care of my Mom but he still wants me home to see him too! So, when I am home I try my best to have quality time with my husband, daughter, son-in-law and the grandkids. All of our friends understand what is happening and send their well wishes often.

When I'm at Mom's and my daughter calls or sends me a text my Mom says, "No you can't have her!" She says this over and over while she's laughing. She knows they miss me and jokes about everyone needing me!

When I get to Mom's the following week I asked her if she wanted to go outside to smoke. She knows smoking isn't helping with her breathing problems. She has been smoking since she was sixteen and feels it's too late to quit now. When I asked her if she wanted to go outside she said, *"No, I haven't smoked since you left last week so I guess I quit."* "REALLY, I can't believe it!" Never in a million years would I think she would quit smoking now, but she has. I told her I was so happy that she quit and asked her how she was doing and she said, *"I'm not going any crazier than I have been for the last couple months."*

She makes me laugh! She's been taking the anti-depressant medicine daily and it seems to be helping her with the anxiety. We went on through the day and I told her later that I thought she sounded like she was breathing better and not getting so short of breath. She agreed that not smoking has helped her.

- If you smoke, try to quit as soon as possible!
- The sooner is better. For most, the first month after you quit smoking it causes you to cough up quite a bit of phlegm even if you're healthy. With this disease it's worse. Mom is breathing better but she is coughing quite a bit.

Mom wanted to take a shower so Dad and I decided to help her. The last shower she took by herself was really hard on her so it's time we help.

Showering Mom:

Mom prefers me helping her. She says I 'know' how to do it better and am a little more careful! Her left arm has no use and she can't walk at this point. She can stand but isn't able to walk. Dad converted the bathtub to a walk in shower with many bars to hold on to. I wheel her in the bathroom on a free standing potty chair with wheels. Help her stand up and have her hold on to the bar with her good hand.

I put a wash cloth on the shower floor so she won't slip. I help her lift her legs into the shower one at a time, very slowly. Then she sits on the shower seat which has a back to help secure her when sitting. She holds on to the handicapped bars at all times and leans on me until she is comfortably seated.

There are many types of shower seats to choose from. If the patient is able to lift their feet, a good one to choose is one that slides from one side to the other. They also need to be able to sit without falling. I put a towel on the shower seat for comfort. I turn the shower on while directing it to the side of the tub so it doesn't hit her until the temperature is safe and comfortable.

Hair first; I use free and clear shampoo and body soap because Mom has a hard time breathing if there's any type of perfume or smell around her. She absolutely loves her hair scrubbed and moans with such delight. She tells me it feels so good! I use a shower scrubber to scrub under her arms and breasts thoroughly. If hands are cupped tight they need to be cleaned really well because they get sweaty and smell. You have to be very careful not to open the hands up because it may hurt. I slide a wash cloth into the curled hand and pull it through slowly.

Then I stand her up, of course, I get very wet in the process but I don't care. I will do anything to help her feel better. I simply stand in the shower with her and keep my clothes on. Once she stands up, has a good hold on the bars, and her feet are stable (I put a wash cloth under her feet to help secure her), I start to clean her legs and private areas thoroughly.

It's good to use a glass of water to help rinse the body. Vanity certainly goes away when you're dealt with something like this. Mom was so embarrassed at first but I kept explaining that it's all natural and that she wiped me all over when I was young! She laughs and is more comfortable about it. She's so glad I'm available and that I'm a girl, she says I understand what needs to be done.

When she's finished I help her stand up and hold on to the bars that Dad had installed. I help her move one leg out of the shower slowly on to the rug and then the other. I hold her body to help her sit in the chair with wheels. Once she is securely in the chair I put a few towels around her hair and body to cover her up and then wheel her to the bedroom to dry and dress. She's exhausted after a shower but feels so good.

The following week:
Wow, it is absolutely amazing how much better Mom is breathing!

- **Quit smoking now! It has made a huge difference in Mom's breathing.**

Chapter 9

The Fifth Month after the Diagnosis

November 2010:

I talked to my California brother about how much worse Mom was getting. I told him that he needed to visit as soon as he could if he wanted to see Mom when she was still able to talk. I'm so glad he listened and made his flight arrangements right away. It was so nice to see him, and Mom was very happy. He handled it pretty well considering he hasn't seen her in about five years.

When my husband and I picked my California brother up to take him back to the airport it was just as sad as when my Vegas brother left. Everyone had tears in their eyes when we were leaving with him and it was horrible driving away. It breaks my heart when Mom and Dad's eyes are filled with such sadness for their family. On our drive home my brother said, "Wow, I can't stop crying, this is terrible." I told him it was alright and that I cry every week when I drive home from their house.

I'm back and Mom's house the next day and Mom is having a very difficult time moving her left foot. It's getting harder and harder for her to move from her bed, to the wheelchair, to her lift chair, and back to the wheelchair. Dad sits her up in bed and moves her to the side of the bed to dress her, wash her, and get her ready to move to her wheelchair.

I don't know what we'll do when she can't move at all but we will figure it out. God somehow gives us the answers and helps us as we are caring for her. She is laughing so much these days. I know that uncontrolled laughter and crying is part of the disease so I take it in stride and laugh with her. Dad has her laughing all the time! It's much better to see her laughing then crying that's for sure. I love them so much and thank God everyday for them.

Thanksgiving weekend:

The holidays are going to be difficult this year since Mom's health is deteriorating and we have to accept that this may be the last year we have with her. Our Holidays were always so blessed and joyful. The girls would go shopping the day after Thanksgiving and Christmas but this year will be different. We would always have a huge toast to our health and happiness, and everyone was smiling especially Mom, with that beautiful smile.

There won't be any big celebration this year, no big toasts to our health, no giving thanks to what we are thankful for, no hugging, laughing, and joking around. It's very difficult to celebrate the holidays when Mom is living her last few months of life. I'm so sad but will get through this holiday weekend and all the others to come.

My daughter had Thanksgiving dinner with our family and her husband's family. This is the first year that Mom and Dad aren't here to celebrate with us and I try to be as joyful as I can. My daughter knows I'm thinking of Mom during the day and touches my arm often to let me know she's also thinking of her Grams. My son-in-law leads us in prayer. I secretly thank God for giving us life everyday and to help Mom live the remainder of her life without pain.

Life will never be the same.

I went to Mom's the day after Thanksgiving and see that Dad got a wheelchair lift for the van. We decided it was time to get Mom out of the house. She was frightened because she had not been out of the house for a few months, but we got her to agree. It certainly took some coaching, comforting, and constantly telling her she would be fine but we did it!

I wanted her to see the Christmas lights downtown since they decorate like Charles Dickens and she would love them. We get her showered and dressed. This is also the first time she's had actual clothes on for a few months. Seatbelt connected on the wheelchair and I rolled her down the ramp on to the wheelchair lift. It worked great! It automatically lifted her up to the van door and I pushed the chair in and got in the van myself.

I positioned the chair and sat in the back seat of the van so I could help comfort her. Once we got moving she was very excited and enjoyed it. She was smiling and saying, "*This isn't too bad and I really like it. I could do this again.*" (We didn't know at the time that this trip would be the first and last time she went for a ride in the van). It was so nice to see her happy. We drove through town and she loved it.

We also went to Denny's to get take-out. Mom loves scrambled eggs with potatoes and veggies. We came home, got her out of the van, into her lift chair and she enjoyed her meal. She's no longer eating at the table because it takes too much strength to move from her chair to the table.

Taking mom out to town is one of the last great memories with her! Enjoy every day that you can!

Mom is still eating with her right hand but it's getting a little slower and difficult because her arm is starting to weaken. I cut everything up into small pieces so that she can pick it up easily with her fork or spoon. Having a bib is a big help. She laughs about it and says, "Don't forget my bib!"

We laughed about me bringing her a cup with a lid and a bib, like you would for a child.
But these are the things that you need when they still want to eat and drink themselves. It's difficult to watch her eat and drink because she's having a hard time. She handles it pretty good though and says, *"At least I'm not spilling my coffee anymore."*

- **Use a Toddler cup so that there are no spills**
- **Bibs help protect their clothes**

Chapter 10

The Sixth Month after the Diagnosis

December 2010:

I broke the news to Mom and Dad that my husband is taking me on vacation from December 3rd to December 10th, and I wouldn't be back to their house for ten days. Mom was sad but she understood and told me to hurry back. She kept asking me when I would be back and I had to keep telling her she would be fine.

My sister would be here for about four days, Mom's sister would be coming to visit and Dad is always here. She seemed fine when I left and I cried most of the way home with fear that something may happen. But I have been away from my husband so much and really think I need to relax and spend some time with him.

Dad tells me that I shouldn't be at their house as much as I have been. He thinks I should be home with my husband and the grandkids but he really does need me. He needs to rest when I'm at their house. I feel so good that I'm able to help as much as I do. I actually feel honored to be helping with Mom's care, and I'm learning so much about healthcare for the terminally ill, not to mention appreciating every day of being alive.

My husband and I go on vacation to the Dominican Republic. Three days after we get there, I get a text message from my sister that Mom is in the hospital with a blood clot in her leg.

*"**Oh My Gosh**, **Oh My Gosh**, I'm so far away. What am I going to do? Why did I leave and should I go home right away? How is Mom? Tell her I'm sorry I'm not there, I'll come home right away."*

I had a feeling something like this might happen. Mom seemed fine when I left but she probably hasn't moved her legs around enough and the blood clot formed. My sister noticed that Mom's leg was really red and swollen and told Dad they better call 911. Mom didn't want to go to the hospital but there was no choice. She worried that they wouldn't be able to pick her up. She thinks she is so heavy. (After I got home she was telling me about it and said they just picked her up like it was nothing!) She stayed in the hospital all week.

This worked out fine since I was away and I worried about Dad taking care of her. It absolutely broke my heart and I was thinking about coming home. My sister assured us that Mom was doing fine and we should stay and relax. On Friday Mom came home from the hospital and we came home from vacation. I went to Mom's on Saturday and decided then that I would never leave them again!

I felt terrible that I wasn't home when this happened and I'm not sure I will ever get over it. How could I leave her when I knew how sick she was? She was feeling pretty good and I knew my sister would be there to help Dad.

My family and friends kept telling me I needed to get away from everything for awhile and take some time to relax. We didn't know how long we would be caring for Mom and I was traveling back and forth to Mom's house every week and did need some time to myself. But, I felt like I had abandoned her.

I was out of the country when my Grandma passed away and I was on a cruise when my Mom had a blood clot about ten years ago (from a routine heart catheter). So, if anyone is sick or not doing well, I won't be going anywhere in the future. When things like this happen, I feel so guilty for not being available.

I went to Moms on Saturday and went straight to the bedroom.

Oh My Gosh, This can't be Mom. I could not believe what I saw when I walked in! How can someone deteriorate this much in one week?

Mom has a new hospital bed. Dad has a twin bed and the beds have been moved around. Now the beds are separated and moved to the other side of the room. Hospice is now involved and they brought the new hospital bed. The beds are separated so that they could get to Mom from all sides without any trouble. Mom looked ten years older and sicker than I have ever seen her. Her left arm had already lost all use and now she isn't able to use her right arm or hand.

This is so sad. How do people get through this with their families? I am dying inside and wonder how I'm going to help her. Her eyes are so dark and sad.

Dad said that Hospice started getting involved when Mom was in the hospital. They told him that they will be here to help us every week.

After Mom got home from the hospital yesterday she started feeling sick to her stomach and had the stomach flu all night. Dad said that she was vomiting all night. I could hardly contain myself. I'm hugging her and she is moaning that she is so sick. She stared at me with those empty sad eyes that say, "Please help me."

I thought she was dying right then and there and my heart broke for her. I can hardly stand to see her in pain and the stomach flu is about the worse. With everything else going on why does she have to go through this? I was wondering how she would even make it another day. She had dark circles under her eyes, her cheeks were sunken in, and she was so sick to her stomach.

Dad was talking to me when I was rubbing Mom's arm and I couldn't hold it in any longer and just started crying. The pain in my heart was excruciating and tears ran down my face. I try not to cry when I'm around them but this broke me up. He said, "What's wrong?" and I said that she looks so sick and I felt so bad that I wasn't here when she went to the hospital.

Mom kept looking at me with those dark sad eyes and I wasn't sure I would make it through the day another minute without totally breaking down.

Her voice was weaker and quieter and she couldn't talk very well. It was hard to understand what she was trying to tell me. She looked so small and was weaker than ever.

As I sat with Mom I was wondering if we had everything ready for the funeral. Did Dad and I do everything we could to help her and does she feel alone? I knew I wasn't going to be able to go on for too much longer so I told Dad I needed to run to the drug store for a few things. I'm wondering how families get through days like this. I'm driving to the store praying to God to give us the strength to help Mom.

On my way to the store I called my husband and cried and cried. I needed to do that so I could maintain a decent composure when I got back to Mom's. He helps me get through these moments by listening and telling me how much Mom appreciates me being there. I get back to my parents house and feel better but still feeling so sorry for Mom.

My Aunt and Uncle called later that day and Dad asked them if they wanted to talk to me, *"**Oh no! I can't'**,* but he gave me the phone anyway. I went to the other room to talk to my aunt and I started crying. I knew I would since I had been pretty upset about seeing Mom in such a desperate state of helplessness. I felt so bad about crying and she tried to comfort me.

Everyone understands what I'm going through and they are so supportive. I try not to cry when I'm talking to family and friends because everyone is hurting for Mom and I don't want to get them anymore upset than they already are.

I can't get over how sick Mom looks.

Mom had been in bed since she went to the hospital and I'm worried that she won't be moving out of bed anytime soon. I told Dad that he should sleep in the spare room so he could get some rest and I would sleep with Mom. He was up the whole night with her last night and he looked exhausted. He has a bad back and was really hurting from helping move Mom around. He said she vomited all night and neither of them got any sleep. She was still vomiting that next night and it was just as horrible.

It took all her energy to cough and vomit, and her breathing was getting shallow. I could tell she was horrified of what was happening to her. She looked at me with her sad eyes as if to say that she needed me to help her get through this. I did everything I could to comfort her.

We did get through the long night and she started feeling better the next day. She started eating little by little. I made some chicken and noodles and pushed her to eat and drink as much as possible.

The bad thing is that my Dad, my Brother and I got the stomach virus and vomited for two more days! I was so sick but still took care of Mom. She can't do anything now so I had to feed her, give her medicine, help her drink liquids, put her on the bed pan, change the sheets, and move her around. She's lost the use of her right arm now and her left leg. She can't feed herself or even move around.

I think being in the hospital with the blood clot and the stomach flu took all the energy she had left and deteriorated the remaining muscles in her arms and legs. We need to move her every few hours to keep her a little active and to make sure she doesn't get any bed sores or blood clots.

- **Once the patient is confined to bed they must be moved often to ensure that no bed sores or blood clots from.**

Mom has been coughing quite a bit and coughs up phlegm that she can't get up. She starts choking on it and it scares me as much as it does her. It's so difficult to watch because it's hard to figure out what to do to help. I use Kleenex to keep wiping her mouth and tongue while trying to pull some of the phlegm from her mouth. She's eating ice chips, Jell-O, and pudding for now.

We started crushing her pills and adding them to pudding so that it is easier for her to swallow. Poor thing, she hates not being able to do anything for herself.

Hospice started getting involved during Mom's hospital stay a couple weeks ago. THANK GOODNESS! The calls started: The Social Worker, the Nurse taking Mom's case, the Aides, and so on.

The Social Worker visited with Dad and I, she is so compassionate that it melts my heart. She gathered all kinds of personal information regarding Mom and the family. She tells us she will come once a month or more if we need her for more support.

The nurse in charge visits with us and tells us she will come in at least once or twice a week to check Mom, take her vitals and help us with anything we need; from changing medication to supporting our sad days.

The aides call and say they will be coming to the house to teach us personal care. When they came they told me they would be coming three times a week to bath Mom and change all her bedding.

Are you kidding me? Hospice will do all this for us?

Yes they will and more if you want it! They are absolutely Angels on Earth! They do so much to help the family prepare for the end; they help with any kind of furniture needs, products, prescriptions, bed pans, supplies, anything! They are so helpful it's amazing!

Our lives have just changed for the better. With Hospice helping care to Mom's personal needs, we have the time and strength to do everything else and most of all, be by her side and comfort her.

Hospice brought sheets, sheet protectors, pillows, pillow cases and hospital gowns. I wasn't sure Mom would want to wear the hospital gowns but she's decided they work really well. She was wearing her silk nightgowns or nothing to bed and the hospital gowns seem to work better since we can leave them untied in the back. The hospital gowns cover her front and she doesn't feel cramped in.

The back of Mom's head has a constant itch to it so she is always asking one of us to scratch her head for her. I'm sure it's because she has her head on the pillow twenty-four hours a day so it gets dry and needs itched and rubbed as often as possible.

She can move her head from side to side but doesn't have the strength or muscle to hold it up for any length of time; it's always on the pillow. Mom thinks it might be the shampoo that we are using on her head even though it's organic, fragrant, and chemical free. We've asked the hospice aides to only wash her hair once a week to see if that will help with the dryness and itching.

I've been trimming Mom's hair every few weeks so that her bangs don't get too long. I haven't been able to color her hair in the last few months so the gray is starting to grow out. She never wanted gray hair but now that she's been watching Kathy Bates on TV she likes the gray and wants her hair to look like Kathy's. We laugh about it all the time.

She's so cute when she wants me to fix her hair and to make sure it's NOT behind her ears! She thinks she has big ears to wants to hide them! The Hospice aides have learned how to fix her hair and they tease her all the time about it. They've become good friends of Mom's and so comforting.

I file Mom's finger nails and toe nails. I also clean her ears and nose when she needs it and clean her teeth every time she eats. I will do anything to help her feel better.

- **Get Hospice involved as soon as possible. They are so helpful it's unbelievable!**
- **Hospice will teach you how to change the bed, move the patient around, massage' their legs or anything that may be bothering you or the patient.**

December 26, 2010:
Merry Christmas

We're pretty sure this is the last Christmas we will have with Mom and it's breaking my heart. We've always had such a great tradition with everyone in the family coming together at my house. We would toast to health and happiness and for some reason we just couldn't do that this year.

My sister and her family came to Mom's, my husband, my daughter, and her family came over with the kids. Mom and Dad just loved being with the boys; 15 months and 9 years. Mom holds a wash cloth curled up in her hands now. The wash cloth collects sweat because all of her fingers are in a claw form. We decide to put the baby on the bed so Mom can visit with him. I put the baby on the bed to give Mom a kiss and he grabbed one of the wash cloths and pulled it out of her hand! Mom has no strength in her hand so she couldn't pull it back. It was so funny and everyone laughed.

These are the good memories! It was wonderful having us together for Christmas at Mom's house, she cherished these moments. I print pictures of all the grandkids often so that she can keep them in her thoughts. She loves looking at them and bragging about each one.

We are also putting a wash cloth under Mom's arm pits. Once the arms start losing muscle they can't lift the arm up and it will hang by their side. The under arm will start to sweat and smell even if they are being washed daily. The wash cloth helps quite a bit.

- **As soon as the patient's hand curls and their arms have no muscle tone, put a wash cloth inside the fingers and under the arm pits. We cut a wash cloth in half for the hands and it fits perfect when it's rolled up. We smooth the wash cloth under her arm so that it's not uncomfortable. Both help keep the hands and underarm dry.**

This disease typically doesn't have any pain associated with it but the one thing that has always been painful for Mom is her shoulders. When the doctor's were initially trying to figure out what was wrong with Mom they thought she had a rotator cuff tear in her shoulder. The pain is similar to a rotator cuff tear and makes sense. With this disease it's actually painful because the arm pulls itself slowly out of alignment from hanging so much. This is the only pain she feels and needs to be careful not to move her arms.

She's taking Vicodin every six hours now and that seems to help ease the pain. We want to get her up and out of bed but we are afraid that we will hurt her arm so she stays in bed. I move her from side to side every few hours and also move her legs up and down to keep them circulated. Her body and legs need moved often to prevent bed sores.

- **If the shoulder is painful when moved, it may help to use an arm sling to hold it in place. We wrapped an ace bandage around Mom's wrist and up around her neck to hold her arm in place. This is something that you should do immediately if their shoulder is painful. We waited longer than we should have.**

Mom's coughing is getting worse and that frightens me the most. It's so difficult for her to breathe when she's coughing and I worry that she will quit breathing all together. She had a really bad spell around 3am.

I sleep in Mom's room now when I'm here so that Dad can get some rest. It's so hard to watch her cough because she gags on the phlegm until she can cough it up. It scares her just as much because she has a hard time catching her breath. She was so upset and started crying tonight. I'm so sad while I'm trying to help her through this.

When she cries she holds her breath and that makes it worse. She wanted me to get Dad but I wanted to calm her down and not wake him up. He gets so upset that something terrible is happening if I wake him up. I kept telling her that it was alright, to breathe, and calm down. I kept rubbing her arms and she finally calmed herself down. She went back to sleep and I sit and watch her for the next hour to make sure she's breathing alright and is sleeping fine.

I talk to the Hospice nurse the next day about Mom's coughing and tell her we need something to help her; either medicine or something to help get the phlegm up. She orders a nebulizer and it arrives the next day. We are now doing the nebulizer three to four times per day and it helps her breath better and seems to help with the phlegm. They also ordered some medicine that helps dry up the phlegm.

- **A Nebulizer is a breathing machine that is needed to help clear the mucus out of the throat. It is also helping her breath better and decreases the coughing.**

I also asked the nurse if she could get something stronger to help Mom sleep better. She's only sleeping about two to three hours at a time and has quite a bit of anxiety again. She's already taking Vicodin and an anti-anxiety medicine so I'm not sure what they will give her. The Hospice nurse talks to Mom's doctor and they order another prescription to help her sleep better.

The nice thing about Hospice is that they are watching Mom weekly, asking us questions about her health, and determining the need for any different medicine.

The Hospice nurse calls Mom's family doctor and they decide together the best approach. Hospice takes care of filling the prescriptions and bringing it to the house. It helps Dad so much because he doesn't have to pick up prescriptions every time she needs something filled.

Mom is still very aware of everything around her and Dad and I talk to her about everything we discuss with Hospice or her doctor. She helps with decisions when we talk about her medicine.

At this point Mom is in bed 24 hours a day seven days a week. I make her tiny macaroni with cheese with chili or spaghetti sauce, pudding, cottage cheese, or soup. She's still using the bed pan with very little trouble. We roll her body over to one side, put the bed pan under her, and then roll her body on top of the bed pan. She hates having to use the bed pan but says it's better than a catheter.

The following week I was on my way to Mom's and my sister called me to let me know there was an incident. She was hoping I was close by and luckily I was. Since Mom has lost the use of both her arms now, she can't help us when we roll her on her side to use the bedpan or change the sheets.

Dad was rolling her over and pulled a little too hard and rolled her onto her stomach and face. She was panicked since her face was in the pillow and her arm was hurting. Dad yelled for my sister and my sister and her husband ran in the room to help get Mom turned over. Mom was so upset and crying hysterically.

When I got there I ran into the bedroom and hugged her while trying to calm her down. She told me she couldn't breathe because her face was in the pillow and she was afraid she wouldn't be able to hold her head up. I felt so bad for her and just stayed close to her side to help comfort her.

I can't even imagine how horrible she feels that she can't do anything for herself. I'm just trying to imagine not being able to even move my head to the side so that I can breathe!

I hugged her and we sat for awhile while she calmed herself down. I asked her if she wanted me to clean her up and change the sheets and she did, she knew it would help her feel better. I changed all the sheets and moved her around and rubbed her legs, back, and neck. She felt better and was so glad I came when I did. She says she was so glad I was on my way and could get there in time to help them.

My Dad felt so terrible but Mom knew he didn't mean it. These things happen and you have to get passed it or you will make yourself crazy. I told him to try not to worry about it, she wasn't hurt and everything turned out fine.

The one thing I've learned is that you take this day by day, do the best you can and make sure they know you love them and care for them. What Mom needs the most is for us to be by her side or not far away.

When I'm not in the room with her I sit in a chair in the living room where I can look over to see if she's awake or needs me. She can see me from her bedroom and I think she has less anxiety knowing that I'm watching over her, even if I'm not in the room.

When I'm cooking, cleaning, or doing laundry, I go into the bedroom about every five minutes to check on her. If she's awake I ask her if she needs anything. If she's fine I will continue doing whatever I'm working on. If she seems restless I sit with her and watch TV or talk to her until she is calm or asleep.

Since Mom is in bed full-time now she seems to have a little more anxiety. She's taking her anxiety medicine every few hours now to help keep her relaxed.

- **Learn how to change the sheets with the patient in the bed. Roll the patient to one side and fold the dirty sheets under the body. Put the clean sheets on that same side and also fold them under the patient's body. Roll the patient over the sheets to the other side, pull the dirty sheets out from under the patient and lay them on the floor. Pull the clean sheets from under the body and finish making the bed. It takes a little practice and gets easier each time you do it. Sometimes I would change the sheets on the days that Hospice didn't come in because Mom felt so much better when her sheets were clean. She also loved her pillow fluffed.**

- **Use Depends or throw-away sheet protectors if needed. Mom was still using the bedpan but we would use the sheet protectors in case she had an accident. She didn't like the Depends and wasn't having any accidents so the sheet protectors worked fine. It's up to the patient as to what works the best.**

With Dad's bad back and bad knee I need to make sure I'm at their house as much as possible. I'm going to try to be at Mom's about five days per week now. I normally come on Sunday and will stay through Wednesday or Thursday. If my sister comes on the weekend it will help Dad most of the week.

Chapter 11

The Seventh Month after the Diagnosis

January 2011:
Happy New Year!

Mom made it to 2011! We weren't sure how long she would live and it's been over 6 months now. The disease is starting to seriously affect her eating and talking and she seems to be deteriorating at a very quick speed.

The worst time will be when she can't eat or talk anymore. I have a feeling it's going to be soon. When she talks I can hardly hear her now and try to read her lips.

We watch her favorite shows daily: The Price is Right, Let's Make A Deal, Ellen and The Golden Girls. Mom also loves old movies that I turn on during the day. She loves to talk about what is happening but it's really difficult for me to figure out what she's telling me and she also tires so easily when trying to talk..

Her voice is a low whisper and it sounds like she's talking in very, very slow motion. Her tongue is losing muscle so she can't form her words very well. I need to start putting words on note cards so she can tell us what she needs with the word choice from the note cards. She's eating ok but the food has to be smooth so she can swallow it. She can drink but has to be careful so that it doesn't get into her windpipe.

I talked to the nurse about Mom's cough again and the problem she is having with phlegm. She brought a suction machine that can pull out the phlegm from her mouth and throat, similar to what a Dentist uses to pull the water and such out of your mouth. I'll probably try to use it soon but Mom doesn't like the looks of it and is worried it will hurt her mouth. I'm sure it will be easy once we get used to it.

I know it has to be better than what we are doing now with her trying to cough the phlegm up and me wiping it out of her mouth and throat with a Kleenex.

- **The suction machine should be used as soon as the patient has difficulty coughing up phlegm. We should have started using it so much earlier. We were afraid to use it but once we started it was so easy and didn't bother Mom at all.**

I wrote down all the medicine that Mom takes and the time for each one. I didn't want to miss any or give her too much so I started a chart to check when we gave her medication. Of course Mom remembers everything and she wouldn't allow us to miss a dose. She needs the anxiety medicine as often as her doctor allows it now.

At this point she's on medicine for water retention, anxiety, sleeping, Coumadin, heartburn, Claritin, antihistamine, and saline in the nebulizer. She takes one Vicodin three times during the day, and two at night, with two sleeping pills. She still only sleeps about three hours at a time though and I'm not sure that will change.

Mom had quite a bit of anxiety this week and coughed so much at night that we didn't get much sleep, other than an hour here and there. I could feel myself getting a little frustrated because I was so tired but I didn't want Mom to think I didn't want to help her.

I make myself think about what Mom is going through. Being a little tired is nothing compared to how she must feel. But then when I went home on Thursday I started getting sick and by Friday I couldn't even talk.

I knew I was run down and needed to sleep. So I stayed home and slept, and then stayed in bed for the next two days. By the time I came to Mom's on Sunday I was feeling pretty good, just a little cough. I know I need to take better care of myself and I need to sleep when Mom sleeps. I'm trying to do too much; laundry, cooking, and cleaning in between taking care of Mom. I want to do it all so that Dad can rest because he is trying to do it all when I'm at my house.

Hospice comes in and bathes Mom but Dad and I take care of everything else. Dad feels bad that I was sick and we talk about it and both decide that we need to take better care of ourselves and spend our energy taking care of Mom, and not worry so much about everything else.

- Take care of yourself!
  - If someone wants to help LET THEM! If friends or neighbors want to help cook or clean, this is the time to allow it. They will feel better being able to help a little and you will feel better being able to spend your energy on your patient
  - Take a deep breath several times a day
  - Get some fresh air
  - Go outside for a walk
  - Exercise
  - Lie down with your feet up for awhile
  - Drink plenty of water
  - Eat healthy
  - Utilize Hospice
  - Share your concerns or sadness with a trusted friend, family member, spiritual counselor, or someone from the Hospice team
  - Get your sleep
  - Take a day off if someone is willing to reprieve you
  - Take your vitamins

January 5, 2011:
My birthday

Mom is twenty years older than me and I'm trying to remember how she was at fifty-six. She was very healthy, having fun, dancing, playing Bingo, playing cards, watching her favorite Steelers play football, cheering for the Earnhardt's in the car races, going to Wheeling to play the slots with Dad, going to Vegas to visit my brother and daughter, going to California to visit my brother and his family, and all kinds of things.

We had no idea that anything like this would happen to our family and I'm so glad that Mom has always been a happy person.

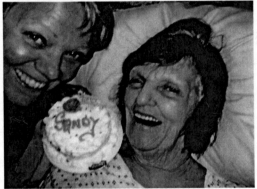
My Birthday Cake! Mom is still smiling!

I'm normally at Mom's four or five days per week and I sleep in her bedroom in the twin bed near her bed so that Dad can get a few good nights' sleep in the spare room every week.

Mom normally goes to sleep about midnight, wakes up around 3am and then 6am. I get up with her anytime she wakes up so that I can move her around and help her get comfortable.

When I'm not here she has Dad move the twin bed next to her hospital bed so that she can be close to him. We were talking about it one day and Dad and I thought it was because she wanted him to sleep near her. She confessed and said that it was because he didn't hear her very well and she wanted him close so he could hear her easier! We laughed about it but I know it's because she has anxiety and wants to make sure someone will help her if needed. She said I hear her every time she moves and it helps her feel better!

This reminds me of when I listened for my children when they were babies to make sure they were safe during the night. It's really no different.

I need to make sure I hear her when we are sleeping; if her breathing changes or she makes small noises I know this is when she's starting to become restless and needs some attention. She can't talk very well so just moaning or making a small noise means something to me. Sometimes I just have to ask her if she's alright and she moans, "yes," and goes back to sleep. She needs that verification that I'm close and can hear her.

The following week, Mom was really coughing and couldn't cough up the phlegm very well. Her throat muscles are getting weaker and it's hard for her to cough like she needs to. She was so upset and that makes it even more difficult. I hate this! It scares me so much because she has such difficulty breathing and I see it in her eyes. She's frightened of what is happening to her and doesn't know what to expect.

I'm doing the best I can to console her but it's just not working very well this time and she's coughing more and more. Anytime she starts coughing I try to settle her down by rubbing her face, arms, and legs. It usually helps to calm her down. Anything I can do to help console her I do.

I know we need to start using the aspiration machine but Mom doesn't want to use it yet. So we will wait a little while longer. I keep telling her that it would be just like what the Dentist uses when he sucks liquid from your mouth. Then I realize that she's had dentures since her early Twenty's so she probably doesn't even know what I mean about the Dentist! No wonder she is worried about using it!

Mom is having a hard time talking and can't pronounce words very well. I'm pretty good at figuring out what she is trying to say but Dad has a hard time so he has me come in to figure out what she's saying. He will look at her and say, "*Jibber, jibber, jibber!*" and they both laugh because he can't figure out what she's saying. It's so sad but they make light of it and laugh. The nurse asked us if Mom would want to use a special computer to help communicate. Mom said, "*No way,*" she doesn't feel like it would do any good and besides, she never did learn to use the computer very well and it would just be too hard for her to learn. I put together a list of words that we can use to communicate. I have been writing down everything she says over the past month so that I don't forget anything. There are several different types of communication tools, but this seemed the easiest for us.

Review the information in www.dynavetech.com to learn about the many different types of communication tools and devices.

Chart We Used With Mom		
Food/Drink	**Health Care**	Bathroom
Coffee	Move Right Leg Up	Turn to Left Side
Pop	Rub Right Leg	Pull Left Arm Out
Yogurt	Pillow Between Leg	Move Up
Pudding	Move Right Foot	Move Down
Cottage Cheese	Right Foot Sore	Fluff Pillow
Soup		Change Bed
Pasta	**Left Leg**	Too Warm
Pasta Salad	Move Left Leg Up	Too Cold
	Rub Left Leg	Wipe Eyes
	Pillow Between Leg	Clean Mouth
	Move Left Foot	Clean Teeth
	Left Foot Sore	Clean Ears

Scratch	Medicine	TV
Head	Heartburn	change channel
Forehead	Vicodin	watch movie
Nose	Spray Mouth	turn up
Mouth	nebulizer	turn down
Chin	drops for cough	
Back	anxiety	
Left Arm	sleeping	Sandy come in
Right Arm		Jim come in
Left Leg		Julie come in
Left Knee		
Left Foot		
Right Leg		
Right knee		

Mom needs to be moved quite a bit now, especially since she's in bed full time. I lift her legs and rub them so that they don't get sore or stiff. It feels so good and she keeps saying, *"Therapy, therapy, therapy," and laughs*.

She has no muscle in her legs and arms and they are getting smaller and smaller. It's so sad to see her shrinking before our eyes. Her eyes have dark circles around them and her mouth gets very dry. Hospice brought Biotene mouth spray to help keep her mouth moisturized and she really likes it. This can be used as much as needed.

- **Move legs around every few hours, rub feet, calves, knees, thighs, and move the legs up and down. If this is not done often the patient will start getting cramps in their legs and feet, and blood clots can form**
- **Make sure to take care of any sores that may appear. Hospice will provide the medication or you can use diaper rash medication that you would use on babies**
- **Biotene Mouth Spray helps a great deal when the patient has a dry mouth. Mom has a dry mouth because of the antihistamine she's using to help dry up the phlegm**

We use different size pillows to prop Mom's legs and arms up, move the bed up and down, move her from side to side, keep her feet resting on a pillow, and have a nice soft pillow under her head. We do this often, especially if she has a difficult time getting comfortable.

It seems like we are moving pillows around constantly. We fold pillows in half and bunch them up under her knees so that she can keep her knees bent. Her legs are extremely heavy now since she doesn't have any muscle in them and they feel like dead weight. When we move her to one side we put pillows behind her back to hold her in place. She likes her knees pulled up and can stay in this position about an hour before having to move her back.

The Hospice nurse has put another mattress made with gel on top of the hospital bed mattress. The extra mattress helps keep her comfortable and help decrease bed sores. Her heels are starting to get sore so we are rubbing medicated skin cream on them and keep them propped up on a pillow so that they don't touch the sheets on the mattress. The nurse said that her heels are breaking down and you can see them turning a purple blue color.

She's still using a bedpan and is beginning to get small sores on her bottom so we are putting heavy medicated cream to heal these sores; similar to diaper rash medicine. It's difficult to keep them healed because of the movement when we put her on the bedpan, but she doesn't want a catheter yet. The nurse brings more medication and a bandage that we can use on Mom's bottom to try to get the sore to heal. I put in on and it will only stay on a few hours since her bottom gets wet when she uses the bedpan. Well, that didn't work so we'll continue putting the medication on very thick to try and keep it dry. My daughter lives in Phoenix and talked to me about what she should do about visiting. She was here to see Mom in August and wondered if she should come to see her now or wait until the funeral. She told me she really thinks she should come after Mom passes so that she can help me. She said that she knows I haven't thought about me but feels I really will need someone here to help me get through the toughest weeks of my life. I told her that I hadn't thought of it but think that she might be right. I told her Mom would be happy that she's thinking of me.

Mom was thrilled that she got to see the grandchildren and great grandchildren in August and she really wouldn't want my daughter to see her now that she's getting worse. I thanked my daughter for thinking of me and thought she was doing the right thing. She talked to a few of her friends that have been through similar situations and they both told her she was right in thinking this way.

She felt better after talking to me about this sensitive subject and I'm really happy. I told her I really appreciated her thinking of me. She says, "*Mom, I know you and you're so strong but this is going to be really hard on you and I really want to be there for you.*"

My younger daughter lives near me and has a nine year old, an eighteen month old, and is ready to give birth to her new child. As much as she will want to be with me she may be pretty busy with the kids. She's giving me the much needed support I need right now. We visit every week when I'm home and I the children help keep me busy. I love both of my girls and their families

My daughters are helping me more than they know. Their loving support is what I need at this time in my life.

I'm so glad I'm at Mom's today. The Hospice aides were here bathing Mom. Dad and I were in the living room when all of a sudden I heard Mom moaning and trying to say something; in a very painful way. She can't speak clear at all and makes moaning sounds but I knew this was something serious. I ran in her bedroom and the aide said she thinks she hurt Mom's hand and was so sorry. Mom's shoulders are very sore since her arm muscles have deteriorated. I held her arm close to her body while trying to get her to tell me what was wrong.

She was so upset and started crying. It's so sad when she cries because she can hardly breathe and then I get tears in my eyes. I asked the aides if they would mind going into the living room for a few minutes while I settled Mom down. She was finally able to calm down enough to tell me that her shoulder hurt when they pulled it out to clean under it.

Once Mom starts crying it takes a while for her to calm down. I rub her arms and face and tell her she will be fine. She didn't want them to think she was angry with them. I told her they were sorry they hurt her and knew she was not angry with them.

The people that work for Hospice are amazing and so strong. They have gone through just about anything you can imagine. I kept rubbing her face and arms and drying her eyes. Then Dad comes in and hugs her and says, "Are you alright honey?" It absolutely breaks my heart. Watching my Dad look into her eyes breaks my heart even more.

My tears start and Mom says, "*I don't want to cry, I can't stop*" and I say, "*I know Mom it's fine to cry, it just makes me cry when I see you cry.*"

Sometimes when Mom cries we end up laughing because we keep asking each other to quit crying so we don't cry. It helps us get through this ordeal a little easier. Once we all calm down I asked her if the aides should come back in. Of course she said "yes" and I went out to get them.

I told them what happened and they felt terrible. They didn't realize what happened and felt bad that Mom's arm was so painful. They hug Mom and tell her that they will be much more careful from that point on. They are becoming good friends and Mom smiles!

The following week I realize the Mom is deteriorating quickly. She is sleeping more and not eating as well. I sit by her side for hours helping to comfort her. She seems so fragile and we try to be very careful with her.

Dad and I were rolling Mom to her side and Dad must have moved her arm the wrong way. She moaned and started to cry and we knew that it had to be her arm. She says that she doesn't want to cry but can't help it. I feel so bad for her and it's pulling at my heart. The tears in my eyes drip down my cheek.

Her eyes looked at me as if to say that she doesn't want to die. My heart aches and I'm thinking: How can I console my mother and best friend when she's lying in bed helpless? I'm not prepared for this. How can I do this? How can I get through this? How can I go on? How can I help her more?

I did the best I could and look her in the eyes as if to comfort her and tell her she will be fine. I hug her and rub her arms, touch her face, and tell her I love her. If nothing else, just the comfort of touch helps us both get through these days. She is helping me as much as I'm helping her and I will never forget these precious days with my Mom. Sitting near her helps keep her comfortable even when she's sleeping.

Sometimes I will go out in the living room when she's sleeping and sit in the chair near her room and watch her as she sleeps. When she wakes up from sleeping I can see her and go to her room to see if she needs anything.

A friend of mine wanted to help and made some Wedding Soup to take to Mom this week. She has been busy with her own mother and new husband but she wanted to show how much she cares. My friends are wonderful and will do anything they can to help me. I pick it up on the way to Mom's. Mom thought it was so nice of her and really liked the soup.

I was feeding her a little spoonful at a time and she was enjoying it so much. Then she swallowed a little bit and it went down her throat and windpipe the wrong way and Mom started choking. She coughed up wedding soup and it sprayed all over her, me, and the bed! She coughed for five minutes; so much phlegm, she couldn't breathe, and her dentures fell out. It was just horrible and I wanted to do everything I could to help her.

She was terrified and I was so worried and thought that she may die right then and there.

I tried to do everything I could by wiping her mouth and kept comforting her and telling her to breathe slowly. I was able to get everything out of her mouth and throat. I finally got her calmed down and wiped everything up, changed the sheets, and her gown, and then told her, "***No more wedding soup for you!***" We laughed together and went on with our day.

It's things like this that make me wonder if I'm doing enough, if I will be able to really help if something gets serious, or should I be asking for more help. Dad is doing great and Hospice is here just about every day but is that enough? I know Mom wouldn't want anyone else here with her so I will continue doing the best I can. I'm not sure my heart can break anymore and I'm so sad for her.

When things like this happen we worry about it but try to get through them as quickly as we can.

- **When someone wants to help let them!**
- **Laugh whenever you can**
- **Always have may boxes of Kleenex on hand**
- **If they have dentures, clean them often**
- **Keep Baby Wipes on hand for all types of clean-up**

Mom is losing weight and her dentures are loose in her mouth. When she eats, food gets lodged in both upper and bottom dentures so I clean them often. If she laughs, cries, or coughs they usually start falling out and I hold on to them until she is ready to have them put back in. Luckily the bathroom is next to her bed because I run them under water every time we take them out of her mouth.

We have a hospital stand next to her bed and it works great. Hospice brought it. The stand holds everything we need: Kleenex, water, medicine, medical gloves, small mirror, tweezers, brush, and a hazard material container for the Nurse to put needles in after taking Mom's blood.

We keep mattress pad covers and Depends under the tray so they are always handy. In the corner of the bedroom we keep the bedding readily available: sheets, pillow cases, blankets, extra pillows, mattress pads, and hospital gowns.

Mom's bed is changed every other day, if not daily. She's fragile but I know she feels more comfortable with clean sheets and fresh pillow cases. On the days that Hospice comes to bath her I have a fresh set of everything ready for them. If I'm not here they know where everything is.

When they finish changing Mom's sheets they bundle them all up and take them to the laundry room. If I ask them they would probably do the laundry too! I feel so blessed to have these special women in our lives.

January 28, 2011:

I went home from Mom's for a few days and some nice good news! My daughter had her baby girl today. I didn't think I would be available when she had the baby but I was actually home and was able to witness this new angel.

The following weekend, they took the kids and the new baby to see their Grams and everyone was so happy that Mom was able to visit with the new baby. It was also very sad knowing she wouldn't be around to watch her great-grandchildren grow up. God gave us this little Angel to help us through the difficult times ahead.

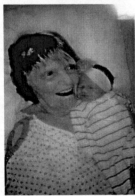

Mom with her great granddaughter and still has her beautiful smile!

Dad had a Bible on the night stand and I asked him when he got it. They've never seemed overly religious in a pushy or aggressive way so it was a surprise to me. He said it was a Bible that was given to him when Grandpa passed away. I've been struggling to talk to Mom about God and having the Bible near her bed would give me the help I needed.

The Social Worker from Hospice called that day and we talked about Mom and she asked if there was anything Dad and I needed. I asked about the Hospice ministry and she said the minister would call Dad.

A few days later Dad told me the minister called but Mom said she didn't really need them to visit since Dad's brother is a minister and he lives about a mile away. Dad talked to my Uncle and he gave Dad a DVD of the Bible. Dad told Mom he was being converted in a joking way and I said, "Wow, that's really cool. We should all watch it next week." Dad and Mom both said we would.

It's then very obvious to me that they have strong Christian beliefs. The only problem is that Mom can only watch a little TV before falling asleep. I will have to see what I can do. I really would like Mom to watch the DVD's with us.

- If you are a religious person, keep your faith and continue to pray. Attend church and stay connected with your church groups.
  - I always believed in God but was never active in a church. I can honestly say that starting a new church during the early days of this experience was the best thing that I could do for myself and my family. I try to attend church every week, pray every day, and feel warmth in my heart that I have never felt before. I know God is guiding me and giving me the strength I need physically and mentally, to help care for Mom.

Chapter 12

The Eighth Month after the Diagnosis

February 8, 2011:

Happy 59th Anniversary to Mom and Dad
They received so many nice cards. Even though
we celebrate we are still sad, since this could be
Mom's last anniversary that she will celebrate.
Dad went to the store and came home with roses
and a card.

We took the roses to Mom's room and she loved
them; then Dad said, "Sandy is going to need to
read the card because I will cry." *"OH Dad,!" I
said, "You know I will cry too, but I'll try."*
Dad laughed and I told Mom that I would need to
read it later because we already had tears in our
eyes. As the day went on I read one line at a
time when I walked past the card.

Mom laughed all day!

We also had to eventually take the roses out of
Mom's room because the smell was too much for
her. We put them on the table outside of her
room so she could look at them all day long.

That evening I felt this strong urge and felt I could
read the card in full, and I did! I read the whole
card without crying and was so proud of myself!

Mom loved it and so did I. She knows how much Dad and I love her and she is feeling the warmth and care we provide for her.

Dad is getting so sentimental anymore. He's always been caring and loving, but now he's showing it so much more with his family. I'm sure he has always shown it to Mom but now he's showing it and doesn't care who sees. He is always kissing on her and rubbing her head and arms and asking her if she's alright.

My Dad is such a terrific, gentle person and they have had a wonderful life together.

Mom is weaker these days and having more difficulty eating anything and especially drinking liquid. She's eating and drinking very little spoonfuls of food or liquid at a time. She's only eating very small and smooth potatoes, pasta, or pudding. We also started giving her a protein drink every day.

Mom likes coffee and the nurse told us that coffee is probably dehydrating her which could be part of the problem with her mouth getting so dry. Mom's probably not drinking more than a cup of coffee a day since it's by teaspoon but Dad picks ups some decaffeinated coffee the next day.

Mom is weaker and is having trouble swallowing food or crushed medicine. When the Hospice nurse comes Dad and I talked to her about Mom's medicine. We asked what will happen when Mom can't swallow at all anymore. She said most of the pain and anxiety medicine comes in a liquid form that can be placed in the bottom of her gums with a medicine dropper. The medicine will absorb into her body. She said Mom will probably stop taking the other medicine for heartburn, water retention, and aspirin.
At that point, it's most important to keep her comfortable. The hospice nurse hugs me often because she can see the sadness in my eyes. I cry while she hugs and comforts me, she tells me I'm doing great and that Mom appreciates all this time she is spending with me. I try not to let Mom see me cry. She has enough to worry about; if I cry she cries, if she cries I cry and on and on!

Dad and I have been talking about the funeral and what plans are already in place. Mom and Dad grew up near Akron, Ohio and raised their family in the same town. Mom and Dad have their grave plots secured and the plan is to have the funeral in Akron, about two hours from where they are currently living.

Dad started thinking about it more and asked me if he should have the funeral in the small town where they live. I told him it's really up to him and Mom; that it might be easier on him if we don't have to travel but he needs to make that decision. I'm thinking it might be easier on all of us if we have it here. It would be a small ceremony with just the family.

He told me to talk to my sister about it and he would start checking the prices. My sister was not happy at all. She said sadly that Mom needs to have the funeral where the family was and that they had so many friends that would want to see her and the family. I told her we needed to support Dad but she didn't understand. She was so sad and we cried softly as we discussed it. She called Dad a few days later and was crying about it because she thought we should have the funeral in our home town.

She was so sad when I talked to her and I told her that we needed to support Dad since it was his decision. She knew that but felt that everyone would be so sad if they couldn't make it to the funeral.

This was the first real tension we've had since this all started and I didn't want us to have a difference of opinion. Regardless of what we felt, we still needed to support Dad.

Dad checked with the funeral homes and asked about pricing for new grave plots. He knew he could sell the plots in Akron if he decided to have the funeral where they were currently living. This went on for a week or so before he talked to Mom about it. He wanted to know the prices and everything that needed to be done before he asked her about it.

He should have just asked her to begin with! She said, "Why would we be buried here when we already have it paid for in Akron? Besides that is where the rest of the family is buried." End of question. Mom will be buried in Akron. My sister was happy and Dad and I were relieved that it was settled. Dad felt better when he talked to Mom but was so sad that the time was getting closer and closer and he couldn't figure out what he would do without Mom.

Valentine's Day:

Mom is having trouble eating but I want to continue trying as long as possible. Every week I've been making a small batch of Macaroni and Cheese, and Pasta Salad made with tiny pasta shells. The pasta normally slides down her throat easily without having to chew it much.

Today it was becoming apparent that eating anything at all would be too difficult for her. I was feeding her some Mac and Cheese and she started having problems eating it. This really starts to concern me because I know that once her throat muscles deteriorate she won't be able to get the nourishment she needs. The Mac and Cheese kept making Mom choke. I told her we needed to stop for awhile and I would try scrambling some eggs for her. It's so sad to watch her try to eat when I know she's hungry and wants something. She's having too much trouble swallowing and is exhausted just trying to eat.

I made some scrambled eggs with soft potatoes and she was able to eat that a little better. Dad also tried a chocolate chip cookie dunked in coffee and she was able to eat it pretty well. She really liked the cookie and it was something different with a little sweetness to it.

We're trying anything to see what she can swallow at this point; cottage cheese, scrambled eggs, mashed potatoes with sour cream, soup, and pudding.

Mom is coughing quite a bit now and having difficulty breathing. Hospice brought an oxygen machine but she really hasn't had to use it yet. I'm thinking we may need to start using it whenever she starts breathing shallow. It's so frightening to watch her go through this and I hate to see her frustrated or in any pain.

Dad and I are talking about Mom and he says, "I can't stand to see your mother lying in bed like this." She has not been out of bed since December and he thinks she is miserable. I say sadly, "The medicine that Mom is on is helping her stay comfortable and she shouldn't be in any pain."

We talk about Mom all the time and he is so sad. He wants to do something to help her and the only thing we can do at this point is be near her side and comfort her. My heart aches for him. They have been married for fifty-nine years and he can't imagine living without her.

Things like this weigh on my shoulders because I want to make sure we do the best we can to care for Mom. I also want to make sure Dad is being taken care of. He works so hard when I'm not at their house and it's all taking a toll on him. He's such a strong man but I can see that he is a little more fragile these days. We can't let ourselves become sick or run down during this terrible time in our lives when she needs us so much.

Dad continues telling me through the following weeks that he can hardly stand to watch Mom lie in bed day after day. He's been talking about getting her up for weeks, even if it's just to sit on the edge of the bed. I'm worried that we will hurt her arms so I'm really hesitant about it.

I buy a large pillow that we could put behind her to help her sit up but I honestly believe that we won't use it at all. Mom doesn't want to sit in bed or get out of bed but she doesn't have the heart to tell Dad. Dad and I talk to the Hospice nurse about getting a lift to help lift Mom out of bed and she's just as hesitant about it as I am.
A couple days later the Hospice nurse told me she talked to Mom about it and that Mom really doesn't want to get out of bed. She doesn't want to hurt her shoulder and thinks it will be too difficult for us to get her up. Mom realizes that being in bed is a way of life until the end.

The nurse told me quietly that she knows how much Dad wants to get Mom up but we shouldn't even try, that it would be too difficult to do without hurting Mom. I told her that I would explain it to Dad. When I talk to Dad he is very sad and keeps telling me how hard this is on him and how he hates her in bed day after day. I told him I understand and feel the same but we need to realize that we would probably hurt her shoulders and that's the last thing we want to do.

We don't want to see Mom in pain or crying anymore than she needs to. He understands but is still sad about the whole situation. He wants to do something to help her and I told him that I think she just needs one of us to sit by her side at this point. She needs comfort from us and sitting with her will help her ease any anxiety she may have.

She's not talking very much at all now so looking into each other's eyes is what Mom and Dad have right now. Dad constantly wraps his arms around Mom, kisses her cheeks and tells her he loves her.

It's been eight months since Mom was given this diagnosis and it's horrible to watch her go through this. I feel so sorry for her that she's battling this disease. I pray to God each day to watch over her and keep her from pain. I still have such a hard time believing that we are going through this in our family.

We've been very blessed and have never had to witness any type of disease with our family members. I try to comprehend that Mom really is going to die soon and it breaks my heart. I can't imagine my life without her, not being able to call her every other day or so to see what she's been up to, visiting her, going shopping together, sharing stories, and celebrating the holidays together. There will be such a void in my life when she's no longer here and I'm so sad.

I feel guilty because I'm sad and feel sorry for myself when I should only be feeling pain for her. My heart is breaking more and more every day. This is a huge impact on me and my life is never going to be the same.

Dad went to the doctor today for his checkup and the Doctor told him to tell Mom "Hi," and that he thinks about her all the time. He said this is the worst disease for anyone to have and it's a shame that there's nothing that can be done other than help keep them comfortable.

The following week I'm trying to feed Mom and she's really having a hard time swallowing, especially liquid. She doesn't want to use the thickening powder to thicken anything so she coughs just about every time she wants something to sip. We started giving her crushed ice to sip on and she has been able to drink that from a small spoon. She likes pop with crushed ice so I give her as much as she wants. That's about the only liquid she's getting these days.

- We are using the suction machine now and it is so easy! I say to Mom, "Why didn't we start using this as soon as Hospice brought it?" She smiles because she knows it was her that didn't want to use it. All you have to do is move the tubing around her gums and it pulls all the liquid and phlegm out of her mouth and throat. She even thinks it's easy and feels so much better. Dad is the one that started using it when I went home last week and said it has helped so much. We put the tube at the back of her mouth and it pulls the phlegm right out. We need to make sure to continue moving the tubing around her mouth so that it doesn't suction and stick to any part of the mouth.

I talked to the nurse again about Mom's swallowing and there is nothing else they can do. It's all part of the disease as the muscles in her tongue, throat and mouth become weaker. The nurse thinks Mom is amazing because she keeps holding on. Her breathing is weaker and she can hardly cough when she needs to. We are comforting her by sitting near her, rubbing her arms, and staying close so she doesn't have any anxiety.

Mom can hardly talk at all anymore and when she does, it's so difficult for her to try to pronounce the words. She is exhausted. I normally try to figure out what she needs just by looking at her. When I tell her what I think she's saying she moves her head a little to let me know if I'm right or not.

She loves to talk about what is on TV but can't do that anymore and it's so sad. She seems very sad these days and I'm sure it's because she knows the end is near. I sit by her side for hours and the only things I can do for her is keep her comfortable and make sure she knows I am always there for her. I would do anything for her.

She knows the end is near.

When I stay I sleep in the bedroom with Mom and Dad sleeps in the spare room. This gives him some time to be alone and get some good, needed sleep so that he can care for Mom when I leave for a few days. It actually works out good because he is with her for three to four days then I come and I'm with her for three or four days.

Hospice comes three days per week to bathe her and changes the sheets. When I'm there I normally change the sheets every day. Mom feels better when the sheets are changed and the pillowcase is fresh.

Every night we watch the Golden Girls at midnight. It runs four shows in a row and Mom loves them. She always liked them when they were on years ago and likes them even more now. We laugh so hard! Mom starts laughing so much that she starts coughing and I worry about her not being able to catch her breath. But she loves the show and watching her laugh makes me feel good too.

I've never been able to sleep with any light on in the room but somehow I'm getting used to it. Mom likes the TV on twenty four hours a day seven days a week. I think she feels comfortable with the noise and that she has something to look at if she wakes up. When she sleeps I turn the volume down but make sure to keep the TV on the stations that air all night long.

She likes the light on but gives me the ok to turn it way down when we go to sleep at night. The TV gives out enough light for her to see me out of the corner of her eye when she wakes up. She can only see me out of the corner of her eye since she can't move her head in either direction anymore.

I can normally hear her right away if she moans or tries to move. I get right up when I hear her and sit by her side. I comfort her while rubbing her arms until she falls back to sleep. I always give her a soft kiss on her face and tell her that I love her when I leave her side.

The Hospice aides normally come around 10am and I always hear them. When they came the next morning I didn't hear a thing and they were knocking on both doors trying to get someone to wake up. Dad was sleeping in the back bedroom and didn't hear them. My brother was sleeping downstairs and didn't hear them.

I must have been really tired because I didn't hear them until I heard Mom trying to tell me something. I woke up and asked her if she was alright. Then I heard them ringing the door bell! I felt so bad and jumped up to let them in.

I told them I was so sorry and we all laughed about it. Mom knows that I'm exhausted but it doesn't bother me at all. I know she needs me. Part of my exhaustion is my concern for her. Mom is on my mind constantly and I'm so sad that she won't be around much longer.

What am I going to do without her?

Chapter 13

The Ninth Month after the Diagnosis

March 2011:

The end is near. Mom's body is so weak and she's losing weight. Her calves are so small from not having any muscle in them but she still laughs about her 'chubby' knees. She says it wouldn't matter how much weight she lost that she would always have those chubby knees. We both got them honestly from her Mom!

Mom is only eating about 100 to 200 calories a day and this will not give her enough nourishment to keep her alive. If she was going to use a feeding tube she would have done that over a month ago. She told me in the beginning of the disease that she didn't want any intervention since this disease had no cure.

She knows that she will eventually lose her life. Dad, the Hospice Nurse, and I talked to her about a feeding tube again but she doesn't see the need since it won't help her get better. It may only help her live a few days longer so she doesn't think it's worth it.

She would also have to go to the hospital in an ambulance to have the feeding tube put in. She absolutely does not want to leave the house. She hasn't been out of the bed or house since December, when she went to the hospital for the blood clot. She does not want to go back for any reason.

Mom wants to stay home until the end and we will do whatever we can to make sure we fulfill her wishes. With this disease, once her breathing muscles quit working the feeding tube wouldn't be any help, so she doesn't see the need. Mom doesn't want any type of medical intervention so we know it won't be much longer. As hard as it is to see her body deteriorating, we know this is what she wants.

It's so hard for Dad and me to see her lie in bed day after day becoming weaker and weaker. Now that she is hardly talking it's more difficult to sit and watch her. My heart aches for her and I pray she isn't in any pain. It's hard to wrap my arms around the thought of not having my Mother to smile with on a daily basis. She is still showing that beautiful smile, even though she can hardly talk anymore.

Mom knows it too. I can see it in her eyes. They are sadder and darker with each passing day. She cries more often these days for no reason. Some of the crying is a symptom of the disease but we also know she cries because she will miss her family.

We make sure Mom takes her anxiety medicine to help keep her calm. We're still crushing the medicine in pudding for her to swallow it easier. She feels better when she takes the medicine and the nurse told me she could take it as often as she needed it, even if it was closer to two hours instead of the normal four hours.

At night she sounds like she has a hard time breathing and Dad is so worried. He thinks too much medicine will hurt her and doesn't want to give her as much as she wants or needs. She gets so anxious and worried if she doesn't take it often.

I keep comforting Dad and tell him that we need to help her stay comfortable and that the nurse told us the medicine is not going to hurt her. He is having a difficult time watching Mom weaken more each day. Even though we've talked about the funeral it's so sad that the end is really near.

March 6, 2011:

My heart is heavy and I can feel the end for Mom is near. Mom hardly eats anything and sleeps most of the time. If she does eat it's only a few small teaspoons of liquid or pudding. I sit by her bed watching her breath. Her breathing is different these days. Her chest wall goes in and out but in a really weird way. It seems like it's going in when it should go out and out when it should be going in. It's so very scary for me and absolutely terrifying for her.

I sit by her bed and rub her arm and face more and more these days. I tell her I love her and that we will keep her safe. I talk to her softly and ask her questions while she moans to answer or move her head yes or no very slowly.

Dad had the Pastor come in and talk to us and pray for Mom. I was so glad to see the Pastor come to the house. Mom has always been quietly religious. Mom has always said that she's a good person, never broke the law, or did anything wrong and that God knows she's a good person. I know deep down, she prays all the time and has a personal relationship with God.

Dad and I have been talking about religion lately and my Uncle gave him some CDs that explain the Bible in detail. Dad is watching those CDs often and I think it helps him get through the days. Even though Mom is sleeping quite a bit now I ask her if we can watch one of the religious CDs that my Uncle gave to Dad.

She motions with her eyes that we can watch it and she actually watched all three short stories with me. I'm so glad she was able to stay awake to watch it and I think it helped her feel much better about what was happening. This was actually the longest she has been able to stay awake at one time.

"Thank you Lord, for giving us this time together"

I go home on Thursday this week with my heart aching, I will be back on Monday and want to spend every waking moment with her from this point on.

DO NOT MAKE ANY PERSONAL DECISIONS DURING THIS TIME OF YOUR LIFE

My heart is breaking and my life is being pulled in every direction possible, *"How am I going to live without my Mom? Have I done enough to help her? Was she happy in these last few months? Was she comfortable? Is she going to heaven? Of course she is. What is my Dad going to do? Should I try to get him to move in with us? Where will my brother live if Dad sells the house? Are we ready for this?"*

I'm turning in circles and I'm not paying attention to my husband, my kids, or grandkids. I act like I'm listening or participating but I don't hear a thing they are saying and have to keep asking them what they said.

I can't remember anything; *"Am I scheduled to babysit or go somewhere? What day is it? Where am I going? What am I doing? How will I help Dad plan the details of the funeral? Will I break down at the funeral? How will I treat my family and friends? What will everyone think of me? I'm the strong one that has been in charge and will I disappoint them?* I'm in such a blur.

Then I do something that is completely out of character for me.

My husband has been so wonderful during the last 9 months and somehow I feel we are having problems and need to separate.

I go to my daughter's house and tell her what I'm doing and she is so sad that I feel this way. He has been a rock for her and she is thinking things will never been the same. I stay at my daughter's house through the day and my husband calls wondering where I am.

I tell him what I'm thinking and that I'm going to stay with my daughter for awhile. He can't believe it and absolutely doesn't understand.

After a few hours, I realize this was a pathetic moment on my part and a desperate plea for someone to help me through this. This is definitely a symptom of the caregivers stress.

I sit there all afternoon and think how stupid I am. There is no way I want to live without him and I'm thinking that I really am going crazy now!

I text my husband a few hours later and ask him if I can come and talk. He sends a text back and says yes.

I realize that this is absolutely not the time to do something so insane and worry that he won't give me a second chance. As I walk into the house and see him my heart cries out to him. We sit at the kitchen table and talk about everything that we've gone through over the years.

We've been married 19 years and have always had a really good marriage. What could be wrong with it? We hug and hug and I cry and cry and tell him how sorry I am and ask him if I can come back. Of course I can! We talk about what happened and what I'm going through with my Mom.

We will never forget what I put us through. What I really needed was more comfort at home and all I had to do was tell him!

As you are reading this, please promise yourself that you will keep communication open with the ones you love during an illness like this. Make sure you ask questions and deal with things honestly. DO NOT do anything like what I've done. It only causes pain that you don't need and it hurts your loved ones. I also didn't realize how much I would need my husband during the following weeks.

Chapter 14

THE END IS NEAR

March 13, 2011:

Sunday:
I was not planning on going to Mom's until Monday this week because of a meeting on Sunday night but when I talked to Dad on Sunday after church I could feel the pain in his voice and decided to go right away.

Dad said that Mom had a really bad night and he couldn't get her comfortable. She was having difficulty breathing and she was trying to tell him something. He could not figure out what she was saying. He put her up, down, rubbed her legs, scratched the back of her head, pointed to words on the word chart, and kept trying to help her but nothing worked.

She was having trouble breathing and he finally realized she was saying that she needed oxygen. Hospice gave us the oxygen machine a few months earlier but Mom never needed it. Once he figured it out he pulled the machine out of the closet and put the oxygen on her as quickly as he could. The oxygen machine has a piece that goes up her nose and wraps around her ears.

I can only imagine how frightened he was while trying to help her and comfort her.

When I get to Mom's she had the oxygen on and I knew this was going to be this week. My heart broke when I looked into her dark, sad eyes. I wrap my arms around her and hug her softly. She couldn't talk and was having difficulty breathing.

How am I going to get through this? How am I going to help Mom further? How am I going to help everyone in the family when my heart is broken? Dear God, please help me.

I tried to feed Mom some pudding but she couldn't swallow. I called the Hospice nurse and asked them if they could bring liquid anxiety medicine right away. She only had pills and I knew she wouldn't be able to swallow them. They sent a new prescription within a few hours. Hospice is so wonderful. We could not have done this without their support these last few months.

Mom is struggling to do anything. She can't eat. She's on oxygen to breathe. It helps that she knows Dad and I will stay with her during this horrible time of her life. Dad and I are heartbroken to see Mom in a lifeless state.

Dad and I realize that her life is coming to an end. We talk about what she has been through these last few months. She really has handled it very well and kept her positive attitude through it all.

We talk about the funeral and the plans we have made. Dad keeps saying that he hates to see her in bed day after day but he can't imagine life without her. They've been married fifty-nine years and have been together since they were teenagers. He doesn't know anything else and I'm concerned for his health in the following months after her death. We talk quietly and try to comfort each other.

As much as I hated to I brought a business suit with me. I had a terrible feeling in my stomach when I talked to Dad and felt that I may need it for the funeral this week. I am so sad I can hardly breathe myself.

Mom is also starting to get mixed up with the time. She slept most of the afternoon and then at midnight thought it was noon. She woke up around 2am and thought it was in the afternoon. This really concerned me and I told her softly that it was the middle of the night. I sat with her and rubbed her arms and face until she went back to sleep. I lie in bed and pray to God that Mom rest peacefully and without pain.

Monday:

The Hospice aides come to bathe Mom and I knew by looking at her that she was too sad to have them stay for very long. I think she knew this was the last week of her life and wanted to be near her family without anyone else around.

The aides came into the bedroom and Mom looked at me and started crying. It just kills me and tears fall down my face. I rub her face and ask her if it would be alright if they just change her bedding and not bathe her. I told her that I could wash her. She nods and I tell them to go ahead and change the bedding.

I normally leave the room when they are with her but today I stay in the room so Mom feels comfortable and doesn't get too upset. These wonderful Hospice Aides. How do they do this? They are so strong. One of the Aides helped care for her Mother during the last year of life and decided to take Hospice training to give back. I could see the sadness in her eyes and knew she was thinking about her Mother. It broke my heart.

The Hospice Nurse told me previously that I would make a wonderful nurse. I've been in the corporate world all my life but I'm seriously thinking about something like this in the future.

The Hospice Aides hug Mom and get ready to leave for the day. They realize this may be the last time they are at our house. I thank them for everything they have done to help Mom and us and I wish them well. I look at Dad and he can hardly tell them goodbye because he is so sad. They have come to love Mom during these last few months and they are very sad leaving the house.

The Hospice nurse came in the afternoon and I told her that Mom was struggling to breathe. I looked at Mom and told her that I felt it was time she put the catheter in. The nurse agreed and I asked Mom if it was alright to put the catheter in. I told her it would be so much easier for her and she wouldn't have to worry about anything.

We have still been using the bedpan and I knew it would be too difficult to continue. Mom nodded. The nurse put the catheter in and it was like all of Mom's worries were gone.

I could almost hear her thinking, "I don't have to worry about this anymore", and went into a deep sleep.

The nurse and I talked quietly about the end of life and she showed me how Mom's legs were starting to discolor, which is part of the process when the body starts breaking down. She said the discoloring normally starts in the toes and goes up through the legs. I asked her how much longer she had to live and she said probably within five days. She hugs me often. My eyes are filled with tears constantly now and I can hardly contain myself.

We have had such a nice experience with the people from Hospice. The nurse would sit with Mom and talk with her about their families for hours.

We had a huge cork board hung on the wall next to Mom's bed with the family pictures and Mom would tell the nurse about every one of her children, grandchildren and great grandchildren. Mom is so proud of her family and loves them all so much.

The nurse has told me several times that Mom is such a wonderful person and can understand why we are so sad to be losing her.

God has blessed me with some kind of strength that I never knew I had.

I asked the nurse if I should contact the family and she said that they should come sooner than later. I cry as she is hugging me and tells me she is so sorry and that she has also loved my Mom.

She leaves and I told Dad what she said about Mom's body breaking down and that we should call the family. He is so sad but says he can't stand to see her in bed much longer. I begin calling the family with a sharp pain in my heart.

My Phoenix daughter is first. She cries softly and says, "Oh Mom, I'm so sorry, I love you, is Gramps doing alright?" I tell her that Dad is doing the best he can and that we will get through this together. She had already told me she would come out and spend two weeks with me. She feels I will need someone to lean on and she wants to be here for me. Leaving her husband and three children for two weeks is a major undertaking but she wanted to do this for me. It's Monday and she makes her flight arrangements for Friday.

I call my Vegas brother and he wants to come home right away. He wants to be able to hug Mom and talk to her before she passes away. He schedules a flight for Wednesday. My husband said he would pick him up at the airport and bring him to Mom's house as soon as his flight arrives.

My California brother is stunned and is not able to catch a flight until Saturday. My heart breaks because I feel that he may not make it before Mom passes away. He tells me to tell Mom that he loves her.

My heart is aching for my family.

How HORRIBLE it is telling your family that their Mom, Sister, Aunt or Grandma is in the last few days of her life. OH MY GOSH, I feel like I'm in some kind of terrible dream. It doesn't seem real.

My Mom's sister has been visiting my Mom weekly for the last eight months and it was breaking her heart as much as it was mine. We cry softly and talk about how much we will miss Mom. Bless her heart. She told me she would call Mom's brothers and my Dad's sister to let them know.

Now it was time to talk to my sister who was already broken up by what was happening to Mom. I was concerned that she would have a nervous breakdown. I have been talking to her since I got to Mom's on Sunday and all she has done is cry.

Her heart was breaking as I was talking to her and we cried for our Mom for what seemed like hours. She lives about three hours away and has not been feeling well this week so it would have been difficult for her to get to Mom's right away. I told her that the nurse said Mom had about five days. She wanted to come right away but she was so sick with the flu that she couldn't. She kept telling me that she didn't know what she was going to do without Mom.

I didn't know how I was going to go on without Mom either. This was something I certainly didn't have the answer to but told her we would lean on each other for comfort. She planned to come to Mom's on Friday but says she will try to come sooner.

Tuesday:

My aunt took the remainder of the week off work and came to stay with us for the day. She is so sad and hugs me tight when she arrives. She sits in Mom's room like I do, rubbing her arms and face while talking about good memories. Mom has been sleeping since Monday but we know she can hear us. She moves her eyelids and mouth when we talk to her.

I sit for hours and watch Mom while I rub her arms, face and forehead lightly. The nurse gave me some sticks that have flavored sponges on the end and I wet them to rub on Mom's mouth to keep it moisturized. Mom is breathing so deep and hard that her mouth gets very dry.

Dad comes in and out of her room and rubs her face and tells her he loves her. She's the same all day and night. Her body is so hot at times and I wipe a cool cloth on her face and arms.

When the nurse comes in she tells me that it's all part of the process. She said Mom will get extremely hot and then cool. She told me she could give her something to reduce the fever but she really didn't need it. Mom was in a deep sleep and comfortable with the anxiety and Vicodin drops.

I could tell when she needed a couple drops of medicine because she would start breathing harder and seemed to be restless, even though she was in a deep sleep.

I didn't want her being frightened about what was happening to her so the nurse told me to give her a couple drops every few hours as she needed it. She never did need morphine. This medicine kept her comfortable and that's what was most important. I would do anything to keep her comfortable and not have any pain.

Thank you, God, for keeping her safe and peaceful.

Wednesday:

We talk to more family members. My brother arrives from Vegas and is so heartbroken. My husband picked him up at the airport and brought him to Mom's. It was so good to see my husband and I certainly needed his hugs and comfort.

Every time someone comes to the house I go through the whole ordeal with them and try to comfort them. I've seen Mom at least four days per week for the past eight months but my brother has only been able to visit two weeks; four months ago.

What a shock it was when he saw her. This is the time when you don't need to hold back the tears. We don't want Mom to suffer but we will miss her so much.

I talk to my sister all through the day and at midnight I talked to my brother in law. He was at work and I told him I thought they needed to come to Mom's as soon as they could. He said he was leaving work right then and they would be on their way as soon as he picked up my sister and niece.

They made it at 3am and once again, the shock and sadness set in. My sister had been with Mom about every other weekend for the past eight months. She knew the end was coming. There is something about being the baby of the family and it tore her apart.

Mom is still sleeping and my sister walks into her bedroom. She starts talking very loud, "Mom, Mom, Hey Mom, Mom, Mom, MOM, Mom, I love you, MOM CAN YOU HEAR ME? Mom, Mom, Mom, MOM." She's crying softly, kisses her, holds her face, and tells Mom how much she loves her. I stand in the doorway to make sure my sister doesn't collapse.

When we go out to the kitchen I told her in a very soft way that Mom could still hear even though she was sleeping. We chuckled about her talking loudly to Mom but nothing helps us feel any better.

I wish there was something I could do to help everyone ease their pain.

Everyone tells me I'm the strong one. If they only knew I was dying a little inside every day. Mom was at the core of everything I did. I got my strength, character, integrity and honesty from her. I've learned so much from her and have lived my life knowing she was proud of me. I've been telling her all along that I have turned into her and she just smiles.

My Aunt told me that Mom cherished all the time I spent with her and that I helped make her feel safe and that I always knew what to do. It has been worth every minute and I wouldn't have changed a thing; I was able to see her at the best times and the worst and was always close to her heart and could feel what she was feeling. She is the example of a classy lady with great character.

During the last eight months Mom didn't want anyone to visit unless I was there. I had a good sense about the situation and could ask them to leave if I saw she was getting tired or anxious.

My niece is eighteen and was so sad to see her grandma in bed during her last days. She was born on the same day as Mom's and that day was so special to them throughout the years.

They celebrated their birthday together every year and I know my niece with miss that more than anything. She asked me if grams could hear her and I told her she could, that she should talk to her and tell her about all the good things going on in her life. I saw her go into Mom's room a little while later.

She was the only one in the room with Mom and started telling her about the musical she was in, and her cheerleading activities. She told me she was so glad she got to talk to her grams like that. It made her feel so much better. I hug her over and over while she cries for her grams.

Chapter 15

An Angel

Thursday:

This was the day. I knew it. I could feel it in my heart. My Dad and I were there. My Vegas brother was there, my sister, her husband and their daughter was there. My aunt was there. Even though Mom was in a deep sleep we talked to her all day long.

The Pastor came and prayed with the family in Mom's room. He asked Dad if he should tell her that it was alright to let go and Dad told him that it was time. Dad couldn't watch Mom suffer any longer. I grabbed my Dad's hand and put my arm around my aunt, my brother held Dad's other hand and we prayed with the pastor.

That was one of the best things we could have done. We all cried during the prayer and when the prayer was over we went out of the room. I felt a great calm come over me. I knew Mom was going to be an angel soon. As difficult as it was for us to let her go we knew she would be safe and at peace.

The Hospice nurse came and checked Mom a little while later. Mom was getting weaker and weaker and it wasn't going to be long. Her breathing was deep and she seemed like she was in a coma state. The nurse talked with Dad while trying to comfort him. She hugged me tightly and told us she would be in touch very soon.

She has been coming to the house at least once a day during the last few days and tried to give us as much comfort as she could. She seemed like she was part of the family now, and came to love Mom.

My aunt and I stayed in the room with Mom most of the day. My Dad was so sad and he would walk in her room every hour or so to hug her and tell her he loved her. We knew she could hear us and sense us being there and we didn't want her to be alone. We would leave when other family members came in to talk to Mom but then would go back in so that Mom wouldn't be alone.

Mom was still sleeping and seemed to be in a coma-like state. I was putting moisture on her lips and cool cloths on her forehead. I wanted her to be as comfortable as possible.

My Aunt and I went to the kitchen around the same time to talk with family members. We didn't realize there wasn't anyone in the room with Mom. We were in the kitchen for about five minutes and I saw Dad go into the bedroom. I knew it before he even called for me.

He called out, "Sandra, Sandra, Sandra." I ran in and knew it. Mom was gone. We hugged and cried and kissed her. I could not believe I was not in the room with her and felt terrible.

My aunt came in and cried, "Why did I leave? She died alone." We cried and cried, "I think Mom wanted it to end that way. She didn't want us to see her take her last breath and she knew we were with her in spirit," I cried.

I couldn't believe this was happening. I must be living a nightmare. It was all a blur and felt like an out of body experience. I couldn't feel my arms or legs. My mouth didn't want to open. I thought I might be going into shock. We all had empty, sad looks on our faces. Can this be real? I know we've been preparing for this day but we can't imagine that it's really here.

We knew there were phone calls that had to be made. We sat for awhile while talking softly about Mom being in a better place. She suffered long enough and her time had come to an end.

She fought the disease well, with so much class, dignity, and a beautiful smile.

We decided it was time to make those phone calls. Hospice had told us that they should be the first phone call that we made. They will send a nurse to validate the death and would call the funeral home.

We were having the funeral in our home town. The funeral home dispatched a driver to pick up the body and would be there in about two hours. Some people would think that it was weird that we decided to keep Mom's body at the house while waiting for the funeral home driver.

We could have had a local funeral home pick her up in the interim but we didn't want that. It was probably one of the best decisions my Dad and I had made! We were all able to go into the bedroom and visit Mom for a little while longer. Yes, she had died but she still looked the same. Her body was beginning to cool down but she was at peace and not struggling to breathe. I was able to hug her a few more times, tell her I loved her, and that I would see her again in the blink of an eye.

I told her to give my grandparents and my aunt a big hug for me. I told her, with a smile, to have an ice cream cone with her best friend from the neighborhood where we grew up. We were all full of tears but there was a nice calm about all of us.

When the funeral home drivers came they told us they would take good care of her. They were very sensitive when moving her from the bed to the gurney. They were careful, took their time, and wrapped a nice blanket around Mom.

They bring her out to the living room and tell us that we can say our goodbyes and they will wait outside until we are ready. This part was very sad. What will we do when they take her away? Our lives have always revolved around Mom, especially the last nine months, and now we need to prepare for the next step.

We tell the funeral home representatives that we've said our goodbyes and she's ready. The come in and tell us they are sorry and that they will take very good care of her. They wheel her out to the van and it breaks our hearts.

Is this really it? Can Mom really be gone? What are we going to do?

We sit around and talk softly for quite some time. We are all trying to ease our pain by saying that she's in a better place now and that she's no longer suffering or in pain. It helps that we are all together but the pain of not having Mom around hurts very much and our eyes say it all.

"And Now She Is Smiling Down on Me And I Smile Every Time I Think Of This Beautiful Woman with a Beautiful Smile"

It's been a month since Mom's death and as I sit and think about her, it gives me great joy to know that I was able to care for her and give her comfort as she struggled with this disease. My heart aches for her and I can only pray that I carry on her strength and happiness with our family.

"I love you Mom"

Mothers Day was so difficult for me. I had tears rolling down my face during the hour service at church and wondered if it would ever get any easier.

It's now been two months since Mom's death and we had our first family function without her. It was so difficult and I felt everyone's pain during the day. The headstone had been put into the ground. We were in Akron for the family function so Dad, my husband and I went to the grave to see the headstone and add some beautiful flowers. It was so much harder than I thought and my heart ached.

Dad had a poem that he wanted me to read and I said sadly, "are you kidding, do you really think I can read this while I cry?" We chuckled a little, he knew I could read it and I did read it through my tears.

Dad is using this poem to put a memorial in the paper for Memorial Day:

In Loving Memory of
Shirley A Gearhart
Who Passed Away on March 17, 2011
We often think of bygone days when we were all together. The family chain in broken now, but memories will live forever. To us you have not gone away, nor have you traveled far, just entered God's eternal home and left the gate ajar.

We Love you and Miss you,
Your Loving Family

- With this disease, there is no cure and you know that death will occur. It may be three, five, seven, or ten years, but it also may be only a few months. One of the best things you can do to prepare is to have the funeral arrangements made in advance. There are so many decisions to make and it is so much easier if you have everything done so that you don't have to go through the pain of choosing everything for the funeral. This will also help prevent excessive sentimental spending.

Chapter 15

My son-in-law's blog

"Hearts Matters"

A Tribute to My Mom

 She had seen it all.....

My wife recently lost her Grandmother. Grams as Jess called her had been sick with ALS for a year. Finally, a few weeks back she lost her battle. As I sit back and reflect on what I knew of Grams, I feel as if I know everything about her because she lives in my wife. I also see the woman she was through my awesome Mother-In-Law Sandy and my wonderful Sister-In-Law Crystal. The reality is I never spent much time with her but I do have a few special moments with her that I cherish. I have thought about those memories as I have honoured her life recently. In this blog I want to share my tribute to Grams.

Here is what I know about Grams:

She loved her family and would die for them

- She has an honesty that not many people seem to understand
- Her will is strong and she will stand for what she believes in
- Did I say she loves her family
- She gets respect from all who knew her

- Laughter is one of her favorite medicines
- Her love language might have been "Acts of Service"
- She loved being appreciated by others
- Humble
- Loved Grandpa and was his soul mate
- In case I forgot Family was the most important
- Appreciated precious moments so much she kept memories, kept a lot of memories
- A one of a kind woman

As a woman who was so loved by her family, I know she loved them as much as they loved her. I could always tell how proud she was of Sandy, Crystal and Jess as I would watch her during our visits to Columbus, Ohio. I would watch her interact with Sandy, Crystal and Jess. It was so neat to see a bond that no one could come between. It's amazing to see her love shine as she lived in the moment with them. I am lucky to have met Grams and I am eternally grateful for her brining Sandy into this world. Then I was truly blessed when Jess brought into the world by Sandy.

One last thought about my mother-in-law, Sandy. Wow, I remember the days Sandy and Grams were visiting Dr. Offices because Grams wasn't feeling well. Then eventually the news came to light of the ALS. Sandy took on an emotionally challenging but beautiful role with Grams. Sandy was there for almost every moment from that point until Grams last breaths. I can't imagine how many titles Sandy has had during this last year for Grams. Daughter, Nurse,

Caretaker, Legal Consultant, Transport
Specialist, Cook, House Cleaner, Estate Planner
Assistant, Organizer, Decision Maker, Life Coach,
Family Informant.....

I could probably go on. Sandy was there until the
very end and even planned her Mother's funeral
arrangements. Can you imagine the appreciation that
Grams felt for her daughter Sandy? She is also a one
of a kind woman.

We all can remember this blog and live as Grams did.
Stand up for what you believe in. Spend time with
your loved ones. Love and respect others while living
with dignity. Listen to your loved ones when they need
to talk. Last but not least laugh darn it, just laugh until
you can't laugh any longer.

Grams you will be forever missed!

Chapter 16

ALS Reference

This reference document will provide information on the symptoms and what you can do to help care for the patient. This information will also be in the order that my Mom experienced each symptom. You or your loved one may experience the symptoms in a completely different order, so don't be alarmed if this reference is out of order with your experience.

- Fatigue: Fatigue is one of the initial signs of ALS. Don't be too alarmed with general fatigue unless other symptoms begin to appear. Fatigue is common in many neuromuscular diseases.

- Muscle Weakness and Atrophy in the arms, hands, and shoulders: Upper motor neuron dysfunction is a loss of muscle strength. As a general rule, ALS patients have little or no pain with the exception of the shoulder. When the deep muscles being to lose strength in the arm and hand a few things may occur:

- o Claw hand is common with ALS and occurs because of the weakness and atrophy in the muscles of the hand and the hand bones. When this occurs and the hand is in a constant curl, begin rolling a small wash cloth to put into the base of the hand. This will keep the hand cleaner, lessen the smell and decrease the sweat. We cut a wash cloth in half and it seemed to be the perfect fit.

- Shoulder pain: This is the only pain that my Mom experienced with ALS. What happens is that abnormal muscle atrophy develops quickly in joints that have little or no movement. The shoulder can also become partially separated or dislocated from the muscle weakness and the joints loosening. This can cause severe pain when the shoulder or arm is moved.

This was one of the first symptoms with my Mom and the doctor checked her for a rotator cuff tear in the shoulder. The symptoms are very similar. Physical therapy to rotate the arm and shoulder around may help with the pain. If they don't want to or won't do any physical therapy, a sling works well to keep the arm close to the body without much movement.

○ Spastic Bulbar Palsy: When the motor neurons and the fibers that control chewing, speaking, and swallowing are affected, the voice may sound forced, very slow, slurred, or quiet because so much effort is needed to force air through the upper airway. Spastic Bulbar Palsy may also cause the patient to have spontaneous crying or laughter.

- Talking: When the muscles involved in sound and speech are affected, the vocal cords begin to paralyse and the voice will have a hoarse or whispering affect and may have a nasal tone. One the stages of ALS as it advances is that it will become difficult to understand the patient for awhile and then not at all.

There are several things that can be done to assist with communicating: alphabet boards, picture boards, word boards, and high technical communication devices similar to computers, a fiber optic infrared switch that is used in conjunction with the movement of the eyes blinking, or an electronic eye-gaze system.

Communication options should be discussed with your speech therapist to determine the best method for the patient. My Mom was not interested in having a speech therapist or any kind of computer so I made my own word board based on common requests or discussions that we had with Mom.

- Chewing and Swallowing: When the tongue and throat muscles begin to weaken, it may become more difficult to swallow. One thing that helps with swallowing, and to avoid choking, is to have the patient tuck their chin down to their chest while swallowing. This helps open up the airway to swallow easier.

  Also, swallow often and take sips of water between swallowing. If you work with a speech therapist, they will determine which foods to eat so that the patient is not swallowing foods into the airway. If you don't work with a speech therapist, you will know when it's time to begin changing to a softer food diet. You may want to discuss a feeding tube with the Hospice nurse.

Hospice does not cover the feeding tube procedure. Work with Medicare and your secondary insurance company to see what they would cover for this procedure. Also discuss this with Hospice because the patient may not qualify for hospice once this a feeding tube is put into place. A feeding tube will ensure that the patient is receiving enough vitamins and minerals.

o Slurred Speech: Weakness of the tongue, throat muscles, and lips may cause slow, slurred, or strangulated speech. As stated previously, there are different methods of communication that can be used to assist the family and caregivers with communication.

o Jaw Clenching or Quivering: This is a normal process when the patient is anxious, yawning, cold, or sometimes when they are speaking. The hospice nurse may recommend a medication that could help limit this problem.

- Laryngospasm

    - The sensation of being unable to breathe or a feeling that your throat is constricting may be triggered by smoke, strong smells, alcohol, or spicy foods. My Mom experienced this quite a bit and we had to be very careful to not wear perfume or clean the house and clothes with anything that had a smell to it. We changed all cleaning and laundry soap to 'free and clear' of all smells and chemicals.

    - Once Mom quit smoking this problem decreased quite a bit. The patient can help themselves when this happens by breathing through their nose when swallowing. They can also apply a few drops of Liquid medicine under their tongue; which will normally stop the spasm.

        You Doctor will determine what medicine works the best. Mom also took a prescription heartburn medicine daily to prevent heartburn; which can cause a spasm.

- Thick Phlegm

    o When coughing is no longer productive, and liquids have been decreased, thick phlegm may begin to get stuck in the back of the patient's throat. The hospice nurse recommended medication will help decrease the amount of phlegm for my Mom.

    Hospice also brought a nebulizer to use two to three times a day as needed. The nebulizer is a breathing machine that helps break up the phlegm; you put a mouth piece in the patient's mouth, add medicine to the machine and turn it on.

    The patient breathes in the medicine for about ten minutes, until the liquid is completely gone. We use the nebulizer every six hours to help prevent phlegm. Even if Mom wasn't coughing or having any spasm attack we still had her do the nebulizer. If we would stop doing the nebulizer for a day or so we could really tell the difference and her coughing would increase.

- Depression/ Anxiety

  - It is only natural that ALS patients have quite a bit of anxiety or seemed depressed. We found that Mom experienced the most anxiety at night when she was laying down. She told me that she was afraid she wouldn't wake up or wouldn't be able to get up if she couldn't breathe.

    Dad would move close to Mom at night to help her feel comfortable. When he got the hospital bed and a twin bed he would move the twin bed next to Mom's at night to be close to her. Mom felt better when Dad was close to her.

    Make sure you discuss any depression or anxiety with the patient's doctor or nurse, so that anxiety medications can be prescribed. This medicine helped my Mom tremendously.

- Fasciculation's or Muscle Cramps

    o These are rapid, fine, flickering, or twitching a portion of the muscles. When the patient has the nerve studies completed, the doctors may ask them if they have noticed and twitching in the arms or legs.

    When electrical discharges of the motor neuron nerve fibers are produced, you may see the legs or arms 'jump' at anytime. Muscle cramps are also common and can occur anywhere on the body; arms, hands, thighs, calf, abdomen, neck, tongue, and jaw.

Visit www.noahbenshea.com Noah Ben Shea is dedicated to sharing his compassion to help others through these difficult times in their lives. He has been named the ALS Association National Laureate.

Reading his information helped me through those most difficult times and my discussions with him on email were informative, compassionate and sincere in wishing us well.

Nearing the end of death:

As part of the dying process, the following is a list of insights, personal growth, and inner feelings that the patient may feel or communicate:

- Sense of completion with worldly affairs and relationships within the community

- Sense of meaning about life and acceptance of the finality of life

- Experiencing love of self and others

- Sense of completion in relationships with family and friends

- Surrendering to unknown, 'letting go'

Withdrawal

It is common to withdraw from friends, family, and the world around them as they near the dying process. The patient may want to stay in bed all day, spend more time asleep, and communicate less.

Touch becomes more meaningful. They may seem unresponsive which is all in preparation for letting go. What you can do to help:

- Plan for visits and activities when the patient is most alert

- Speak to the patient in a normal tone. Hearing remains intact to the end

- Tell the patient what you are going to do before you do it: giving medicine, combing hair, changing sheets, preparing food, feeding them, etc.

- Do not say anything in front of the patient that you wouldn't say if they were awake. They can normally hear you even while sleeping

Changes in Appetite

The patient will eventually no longer be interested in food or they may become unable to eat or drink. Because eating helps nourish the body this is very difficult for caregivers to accept. Weight loss will be expected. What you can do:

- The patient will let you know if they want food or fluids. Often with ALS this will be determined by what they can or can't do

- Liquids will be preferred to solids. Crushed ice or a Milk Shake made with a protein drink seemed to help Mom stay hydrated

- If the patient is not able to speak they will let you know if they are finished by closing their mouth or, if they can, turning their head to the side

- Don't try to force the patient to eat or drink. Respect their wishes. Use a swab dipped in water to wipe their mouth and lips to help keep moisture on the lips

Changes in Elimination

As a patient declines the urine output usually diminishes and the color is usually darker than normal. It may also have a strong odor and appear cloudy. What you can do to help:

- Adult disposable briefs and under pads on the bed may help solve some of the problem. The nurse or home health aide will show you how to change these for the patient that is confined in bed

- Once the patient is bedridden, it may be appropriate to use a catheter. The catheter will help keep the patient's skin dry

- There are also certain medicated lotions and creams that the nurse will recommend you apply periodically to the patient. If you don't get the medication from your nurse you can use diaper rash medicine that would be used for a baby

- To help maintain dignity make sure you provide privacy when changing the bed or providing personal care. Check the patient frequently to ensure that they are kept dry and comfortable

Changes in Breathing

When the patient is nearing the end their breathing patterns often begin to change. Their breathing may become rapid, slow down, shallow, or short periods of no breathing which can last up to a full minute. This is not uncomfortable for the patient but you should talk to the nurse to see if oxygen is needed.

When an ALS patient is having difficulty swallowing, saliva gathers in the back of the throat that may make a rattling noise. It may be concerning but does not necessarily indicate that the patient is suffering. What you can do to help:

- Turning the patient on their side or raising the head may assist to drain the secretions

- The patient's nurse may also prescribe medication that can dry excess secretions

- The patient will probably be breathing with their mouth open. This dries the mouth out and the nurse may prescribe Biotene, which is a good treatment that will help moisturize the mouth

- Once breathing becomes difficult for the patient the nurse may prescribe an anxiety medication that will help keep the patient comfortable

Changes in Body Temperature

Fever

As the body becomes weaker the patient may have a fever or their temperature may drop and cause the body to become cool. Sometimes the patient may become sweaty and clammy with or without a fever. What you can do to help:

- Let the nurse know if the patient starts developing a fever. They may recommend Tylenol to help reduce the fever. Placing a cool cloth over the forehead and removing blankets may help

- Open the window for cool air or use a fan

- The patient may feel cool but could be warm on the inside. If they want the blankets off, take them off, even if they feel cool

    o To help keep Mom comfortable, we were often taking blankets off and putting them back on

Coolness

As the patient becomes weaker their circulation decreases. You may notice that they feel cool to the touch. Their hands and feet may become purplish, and the knees, ankles, and elbows may look blotchy.

The patient may appear pale and have a bluish cast around the lips and under the fingernails. The patient isn't in any discomfort as it is a natural part of the dying process. What you can do to help:

- Use a warm blanket but not electric

- Continue to reposition the patient and provide gentle massages

Confusion and Disorientation

Patients near the end of life may have confusion about the time, surroundings, and who the people around them are. They may also talk about travel as though they were planning a journey.

This may be one way that they are preparing for death or telling you goodbye. What you can do to help:

- Let the Hospice nurse know of these symptoms. They may review the medication or inform you of ways you can provide care and support

- You may want to remind them of who you are and what you are doing while pointing out familiar surroundings

- Provide the patient with reassurance by reminding them of your presence and support

- This may be the time when you limit visitors to decrease the level of confusion

- Do not contradict or argue with the patient. Listen carefully as there may be meaningful messages that they are sharing

- Being available is the most important thing you can do for your patient

Agitation and Restlessness

It is not uncommon for the patient to pick at their bed clothes or perform repetitive movements. This may be due to a variety of physical or emotional reasons.

Agitation or restlessness may be a symptom of discomfort, emotional or spiritual concerns, unresolved issues, or unfinished tasks. What you can do to help:

- Inform the Hospice nurse so that they will assess the situation for any underlying pain or discomfort. They may increase the amount of anxiety medication to help ease the restlessness

- Allow the Hospice social worker and/or chaplain to address any underlying concerns regarding emotional or spiritual support. Your place of worship may also be contacted for spiritual support

- Reassure the patient by speaking slowly, calmly, and in a soothing way

- Offer to take over any tasks or issues that the patient is wanting to accomplish

- Reading an inspirational book or playing soothing, soft music

- Holding the patient's hands or touching them lightly

- Use bed rails and have someone sit with the patient to help keep them safe

- Consider using a baby monitor while out of the room to listen for any signs of restlessness or breathing difficulty

- Share memories of special occasions, holidays, family experiences, or their favorite places

Surge of Energy

The dying patient may have a sudden surge of energy which is normally short lived. They may become alert and clear or ask to eat when they haven't had anything to eat in days.

They may be awake more than normal. It doesn't mean that they are getting better. It normally means that they are using all their physical strength for the last full days of life. What you can do to help:

- Enjoy this time with your loved one

- Say goodbye and reminisce

- Hold hands and gently rub the patients face and arms

Saying Goodbye

You may feel it is not appropriate to say goodbye. You may be concerned that it will hasten death or possibly communicate something unintended. You may not know what to say or have questions about whether you should give permission to let go.

This is a personal decision and there is no right or wrong. You will know in your heart when to say goodbye and how to say it. This time with your loved one is precious and sometimes the Pastor will start the conversation in prayer. What you can do to help:

- Take this opportunity while the person is alert, to say or do what you need to

- Listen to your heart and follow its guidance

- Some conversations begin with

- *What I love the most about you* _____

- *What I will always remember* _____

- *What I will miss most about you* _____

- *What I learned from you* _____

- *What I will cherish* _____

- This may also be a time to say that you are sorry for something, share forgiveness, or let go of past conflicts

- Share your expression of gratitude

- If appropriate, lie in bed with your loved one and hold them or take their hand and say everything you may need to say

- Saying goodbye is a healthy expression of your love and tears are a normal process. Sometimes it can help ease the pain when both of you cry

Reviewing the Symptoms of Approaching Death

One to Three Months:

- Withdrawal from activities and people

- Less communication

- Drinking and eating less

- More sleeping

One to Two Weeks:

- Confusion and disorientation

- Talking about taking a journey or travelling

- Talking to people not present in the room

- Physical change:

    o Decrease or increase in the pulse

    o Decrease in blood pressure

    o Skin may become blotchyr

    o Irregularities in breathing

    o Changes in body temperature; hot or cold

    o Taking little or no fluids, not eating

Days to Hours:

- Sleeping the majority of the time

- Restlessness or agitation

- Surge of energy

- Difficulty breathing or swallowing

- Further discoloration of the skin

- Rattling sounds when breathing

- Weak pulse

- Decreased urine

- Eyelids not able to close completely

Minutes:

- Shallow breaths with longer pauses

- Mouth open

- Unresponsive

  - With ALS these symptoms may last a few hours to a few days

"In this life we cannot do great things. We can only do small things with great love"

Mother Teresa

Moment of Death

It is important to discuss with caregivers, friends, and family what to do if they are present at the time of death. Regardless of how well you prepare yourself, death will still feel like a shock. If you are utilizing Hospice nothing needs done other than to call them.

The Hospice nurse will visit to confirm the death and remove any tubes that are present. They will dispose of medications and call the funeral home if you wish. If the funeral home is in a different town you can do a couple different things; you can have a local funeral home come and take the body until the out of town funeral home arrives, or you can keep the body until the out of town funeral home arrives to get the body.

Your decision will depend on how long it will take the funeral home to pick up the body. It will be up to you if you decide to be present when the funeral home prepares the body for the ride to the funeral home.

Funeral arrangements need to be made. With ALS, there is no cure and you should have time to coordinate funeral arrangements before the time of death. I highly recommend having the majority of the funeral arrangements made prior to death, as it will ease the discomfort when meeting with the funeral director. It may also decrease the unnecessary spending associated with planning a funeral.

God Bless You, Take care

"My wish is that you have learned about the disease and that this personal story has helped or will help you understand what you have gone through or will go through. Take your time with the ones you love, cherish every minute, love them with all your heart and most of all care for yourself."

Sandy Donalds

CPSIA information can be obtained at www.ICGtesting.com
Printed in the USA
BVOW03s1422260415

397752BV00014B/473/P